Hope for Healing
Liver Disease
In Your Dog

The Complete Story

by
Cyndi Smasal

Forward by Deb Forster, B.S., D.V.M.

authorHOUSE®

AuthorHouse™
1663 Liberty Drive, Suite 200
Bloomington, IN 47403
www.authorhouse.com
Phone: 1-800-839-8640

Printed in the United States of America
Bloomington, Indiana
This book is printed on acid-free paper.

ISBN: 978-1-4343-1916-6 (sc)
ISBN: 978-1-4343-1915-9 (hc)

Library of Congress Control Number: 2007904115
Material for this book has been compiled from books I have read, articles I found on the
Internet, and trial and error. I have made every effort to credit my sources. If I have
made any omissions, I will gladly make the correction once it is made known to me.

Reprinted from <u>*DR. PITCAIRN'S COMPLETE GUIDE TO NATURAL HEALTH FOR*</u>
<u>*DOGS & CATS*</u> *© 1995 by Richard H. Pitcairn and Susan H. Pitcairn. Permission*
granted by Rodale, Inc., Emmaus, PA 18098. Available wherever books are sold or visit
<u>*www.rodalestore.com*</u> *or call the Publisher at (800) 848-4735.*

All website addresses were correct at the time of publication.

Legal Notice

This book is dedicated to my companion, best friend and dog Norman.

Contents

Foreword

By Deb Forster, B.S., D.V.M.

*"This is vital information that needs to be available for every
pet-lover who has a dog with liver disease."*

In my 20 plus years as a veterinary practitioner, I've treated many cases of liver disease, and I've followed both conventional and alternative methods of healing. In these pages, Cyndi Smasal has compiled an excellent guide to help treat liver disease in dogs, our best friends and companions. And, it's in a great format that will allow readers to download it off the World Wide Web.

I started working with Cyndi and Norman four months into her alternative treatment. I've never met a more dedicated pet owner. She became a student and now a teacher of alternative veterinary medicine, nutrition, supplements and homeopathic remedies. I have personally seen Norman benefit from her loving care, homemade dog food and nutritional supplements.

The concept of a special diet for liver disease is not a novel one. But in this book, Cyndi addresses the topic from a very personal and truthful level. She has tried everything that could possibly be helpful for her dog, much more than what she's listed in these pages. She's put all the results of her research into an easy to read, concise book that fills a tremendous need in the pet-lover community.

You will find her determination inspiring in addition to solid information about a complex disease. This book is by no means the answer to all of your dog's needs, but it provides a great start for treating your dog with liver disease in collaboration with a qualified veterinarian.

This is vital information that needs to be available for every pet-lover who has a dog with liver disease.

Deb Forster, B.S., D.V.M.
Four Paws Vet Hospital
8401 Ranch Rd. 12
San Marcos, TX 78666
Phone: (512) 396-7297
www.fourpawsvethospital.com

A Note of Caution

The material in this book has been written for educational purposes ONLY. It should not be regarded as veterinary medical advice. I am not a veterinarian. Please consult with a Doctor of Veterinary Medicine or a holistic veterinarian before applying what you learn from this book.

My approach to treating liver disease is considered to be alternative by definition. My approach has not been investigated or approved by any regulatory agency. Do not use this book as a substitute for treatment by a veterinarian. Rather, use this information in conjunction with veterinary care. Always discuss the use of alternative approaches like this one with your veterinarian before trying them.

I did not receive an enthusiastic response from my first veterinarian when I discussed this approach. So, you may want to consult with more than one veterinarian regarding the treatment that is best for your dog.

Ultimately, you are responsible for the care and treatment that your dog receives. I am not responsible for any adverse reactions or effects resulting from the use of the information contained in this book.

Introduction

By Donna M. Hilbig, M.Ed., L.P.C.

I have been privileged to witness the events described in this book, because of my acquaintances with both the author and Norman, the spunky Cocker Spaniel upon whom this book is based. In the following pages you, too, will sense the depths of the relationship between this dog and his human. From the beginning, it was obvious that he claimed her heart, and they belong to one another.

Being a "cat person," it was a foreign concept to hear someone say they have to go straight home after work, "because Norman is by himself." Seeing a dog sit and sleep in a person's lap in the same way a cat does was mind-boggling to me. But all it took was one incident of Norman having an irritation of his "third eyelid" to understand that these two were connected in a way beyond my sensory ability. There were tears of frustration, because Norman was suffering and Cyndi wanted to help him feel better. "He doesn't complain unless he's really feeling bad," she said. I went over to help as she gently rinsed his eye, and he was better. In time, I would see for myself that Norman truly is a very happy dog with a very loving personality.

Norman is also a very communicative dog. He smiles as he pants when he's happy. And he actually "frowns" when he realizes Cyndi is going somewhere but he's not invited. Granted, Cyndi hates having to leave him and has often fantasized out loud about taking him to work with her! So, when he's sick, it's very easy to tell. Norman just isn't his normal, happy, playful self.

When he was diagnosed with liver disease, it was almost as if he had already died. He was very uncomfortable from having a swollen belly, and Cyndi just couldn't stand to see him suffer. Amazingly, the swelling went down quickly. Then, something more amazing happened. The woman I knew as a very skilled Quality Assurance Engineer in the computer programming industry began to approach Norman's medical condition as if it were "defective software." She put her analytical skills to work overtime, believing that there was an eventual solution.

I was a witness to a miracle in progress as she tried one intervention after another. After each effort, she would develop a "new and improved" process. Through it all, Norman's blood tests just got better and better! Today, if it weren't for his debilitating arthritis, Norman would easily be mistaken for a two-year old puppy. He is truly a special dog, and he has chosen a very special human with whom to share his life.

Even though Cyndi is Norman's "provider," he has given her just as much, if not more. Together, they have learned to love unconditionally and to roll on the ground just for the pure joy of it. Norman's philosophy of life is "smell everything, lick as if your life depends on it, wear your heart on your sleeve — then it's easier to get to when it's hurting, always express your feelings, and forgive every time you're asked." Sounds like a great way to live!

Chapter 1 – Norman's Story

"Blessed is the person who has earned the love of an old dog."
– Sydney Jeanne Seward

It was close to Christmas 2001 and something inside me kept telling me that there was something wrong with Norman. I thought the worst. "It must be cancer. He's going to die, I just know it." I finally decided to face my worst fears and take him in to see the Vet. I took him to the same Vet he had been seeing for 8 years. The symptoms I described were: excessive drinking, accidents (overabundance of urine), vomiting, diarrhea (soft stools) and flecks of blood in the vomit. Dr. X did a blood test, came back and told me he had liver disease. I asked what the treatment was for liver disease and he said there really wasn't anything he could do. The next step was to determine how bad and how far along it was by doing an ultrasound. Norman had also been taking Rimadyl for Arthritis pain in his hips and knees. Dr. X. told me to stop giving it to Norman since it could be harmful to the liver. So, I scheduled the ultrasound, stopped the Rimadyl and started feeding Norman a prescription diet food for liver disease.

The next week Norman seemed to get worse. He swelled up like a balloon weighing in at 34 pounds. I thought he was going to pop he was so big. I took him in again to see if there was something that the Vet could do. A different Vet (Dr. Y) saw him and said that the fluid should not be removed and that the body would absorb it. The ultrasound was done while Norman was in this bloated state.

The Vet who performed the ultrasound consulted with Dr. X and they decided not to do a biopsy because the liver was too small, there was too much fluid and the prognosis was not very good. Dr. X didn't see any point in spending more money on a dying dog.

I started taking Norman in to see either Dr. X or Dr. Y every week to check Norman's blood levels.

The last time I saw Dr. X he further diagnosed the ultrasound as Cirrhosis. At this time, I asked Dr. X for prognosis and treatment options. He said he would probably live 14-30 days and that there wasn't a formal conventional medical treatment for Cirrhosis. Just like humans, it was a slow and inevitable death. He said Dr. Y recommended a natural supplement (Milk Thistle) that she believed in but he didn't necessarily offer any real hope. Dr. Y shared with me that the liver is an organ that can rejuvenate but not if it's damaged beyond repair. She ordered the Milk Thistle for me and we started giving Norman Milk Thistle and Vitamin E along with the prescription diet food for liver disease.

I went home and began to mourn over what seemed to be the inevitable death of my 10-½ year old cocker spaniel. I held Norman in my lap and hugged on him like he could die tomorrow; and I prayed to God for a miracle.

"Lord, I thank you for putting Norman in my life. I know it seems silly to pray for a dog, but you know how special he is to me and how much I love him. So, I ask if it is your will, to allow him to live. And if it's not, I ask that you take him soon so he does not suffer. In Jesus' name. Amen."

With my prayers in God's hands, I began to do research to see if there was anything else I could do to take better care of Norman.

Hope for Healing

I started my research on my computer, searching the Internet. I found very little, but I did find one article that gave me hope. It was called Sunny's Miracle Diet. Sunny's story seemed very similar to Normans. Sunny had all the same symptoms, and using a natural home cooked diet, Sunny was still alive after 6 months. This hope spurred me on to find out as much as I could about liver disease, Cirrhosis, Natural Diets and food remedies for liver disease. All the information I found was scattered, and one seemed to contradict the other. So, I continued to search, and purchased all the books I could find on Natural Dog Diets and Natural Dog Care. One thing was becoming clear. The ONLY treatment for liver disease was through a radical change in DIET.

During the time I was collecting my data and doing research, Norman had been on a prescription diet food for liver disease. I started noticing that Norman's love for eating the new food was growing into what looked like a mad starving animal. He seemed to be hungry all the time and was always wanting more and more to eat. This concerned me, but it wasn't until I noticed Norman going to the extreme of actually eating his own stool that I knew this wasn't good for him.

I decided to take a chance and made Sunny's Miracle Diet for him to eat instead of the prescription diet food. I didn't have all the information about natural diets at this time, so I didn't know that it wasn't the "perfect meal" for Norman. But, I thought it had to be better than the prescription diet food.

Norman loved the home cooked meal and seemed to be very satisfied with it. Although I did allow him to eat more than I normally would, I didn't let him eat until he stopped on his own. He didn't seem to want to stop. But, I did allow him to eat several bowls of Sunny's Miracle Diet.

As I started compiling the research and learning more and more about Natural Diets, I found that none of the books really had a "perfect meal" for Norman. I realized quickly that there was no sure-fire "perfect recipe" that I could follow. I was going to have to either hire a Nutritionist or learn what I needed to know and do it myself.

I was short on finances, so I decided to learn for myself.

The rest of this book is a compilation of what I have learned after more than a year of caring for Norman. I include what I have tried, what I have learned, what worked and what didn't. I hope that this book saves your dog's life and gives you everything you need to care for the dog that you love.

I had nothing to lose, and the life of my dog to gain!

Since the Vet told me Norman was likely to live only another 14-30 days, trying a different food couldn't be any worse than doing nothing and allowing him to die. I decided I had nothing to lose, and I wasn't going to sit around and do nothing.

So here's what I did:

1) Stop using Conventional Medications! (Antibiotics, Pain Medications)
2) Start dosage of Milk Thistle (Silymarin) to support the liver (150mg 1/day)
3) Start dosage of Vitamin E to help detoxification (400 I.U. daily)
4) Start dosage of Ursodiol to add Bile Acid to help digestion
5) Start dosage of Multi-Vitamin with antioxidants (1/2 of human Multi-Vitamin per day)
6) Stop feeding prescription diet food for liver disease
7) Start Basic Natural Diet with recommendation for Liver Diet
8) Start using Distilled Water

Three months later, I went in to get a follow-up blood test for Norman. I asked the Vet about the Natural Diet and Sunny's Miracle Diet. She was not in favor of changing Norman to the Natural Diet and stood by the prescription diet food. I told her I had already made the switch and was going to stick to it.

Norman's Blood Test came back NORMAL!

She ran a full-spectrum blood test to see how Norman was doing. I also suspect she wanted to show me some deficiencies from Norman's diet to convince me to put him back on the prescription diet. The results came back that everything was NORMAL. Three months of Natural Diet and Supplements and Norman was back to NORMAL!

Norman's liver was more than likely still damaged, but it was rejuvenating just like I hoped. My prayer had been answered. **Norman wasn't just living with liver disease, he had survived it!**

Once diagnosed with liver disease, you can never fully recover as if no disease had ever occurred. So, it was never an option for me in my mind to stop the Natural Diet and Supplements.

My research continued as I searched for ways to improve Norman's diet.

I continued to find more and more information about liver disease (in humans and animals) and how to treat it with all sorts of alternative treatments, including food remedies. I started compiling a list of all the foods that were "good for the liver" and anything that was "not good for the liver".

Norman's Next Crisis Led Me to Find a New Vet.

Several months into the Natural Diet, Norman started having new symptoms.

Normans new symptoms included: vomiting up his undigested food in the middle of the night, waking me up to let him outside 2 to 3 times a night, having accidents if left alone for more than 4 hours, and diarrhea. At it's worst point, Norman wouldn't eat, and his stool looked bloody. I took Norman in to see the Vet again and she kept him overnight to determine if he was having Liver Failure, or something else. She kept an IV in him with Vitamin B-12 in it all night, and in the morning I was there to feed him his Natural Breakfast. He ate it up and we went home. Norman was better, but he was still having many of the same symptoms. He was waking me up at night, vomiting his undigested meal, and had occasional diarrhea. I was unhappy with the last visit with the Vet. So, I decided I needed some more help with Norman's diet and supplements. **I wanted a Vet who would explain more to me about his condition and give me the support I needed** to improve Norman's diet and his condition.

I interviewed a Homeopathic Vet who did not practice conventional medicine anymore. She opened my eyes to the world of Homeopathic medicine. We spoke on the phone several times, and I tried some of her homeopathic prescriptions to help Norman with his upset stomach. But, the end of this crisis came from due diligence on my part with careful note taking, and noticing all of Norman's behaviors and reactions after every meal.

I began my analysis by taking a scientific approach to diagnosing what was causing Norman's reaction. My hypothesis was that something in his diet was causing or contributing to his upset stomach, gas, diarrhea and vomiting. I just needed to figure out what it was. By this time, I had a very sophisticated diet consisting of a variety of meals and supplements. In order to determine what the culprit was, I was going to have to change only one variable at a time and see if it had any effect on his system.

I did this by sticking to one type of meal all day for several days to make sure that it came out (in the stool) okay. It takes 12-16 hours for a meal to go all the way through Norman's system from feeding to stool. I know this through giving distinctively different meals, then watching and timing when they came out. For example, carrots are not always completely digested. Feeding carrots in one meal and not in the next will allow you to tell when that meal was digested.

For 3 days I made notes on everything that Norman did, when he did it, how he did it and what it looked like. I removed one item from his diet at a time and waited at least a day before removing the next item. Finally, I found the culprit. Rice! Once I removed rice from Norman's diet everything went back to normal again. You must stick with the same meal that works for several days to make sure that everything is truly back to normal.

Here's a list of things to watch and note if you are trying to identify problem foods.

Laying (sleeping) Spots
Feeding Time
Urination Time
Bowel Movement (potty) Time
Stool Color, Consistency and Volume
Behaviors (e.g. sleeping, licking on a part of body, walking around frequently, begging, eating strange objects like charcoal, grass or feces,)
Timing of Behaviors
Meal Ingredients
Supplements Given
Timing of Supplements Given (with or without food and time of day)

Here's an example of one day's notes on Norman.

		Wednesday
	Date	**7/22/03**
MORNING	Wake-Up Time	6:30am
	Morning Med Time	(usual) 7:00am
	Breakfast Time	7:15am
	Potty Patrol Check	Brown, Solid, Normal – 9:35am
NOON	Arthritis Med Time	(usual) 11:00am
	Lunch Time	11:15am
	Ursodiol	(Yes) 11:15am
	Potty Patrol Check	Brown, Solid, Normal – 11:35am
	Lunch Vitamins & Supplements	(usual) 11:15am with lunch
AFTERNOON	Arthritis Med Time	(usual) 3:00pm
	Dinner #1 Time	3:15pm
	Potty Patrol Check	None
EVENING	Arthritis Med Time	(usual) 7:00pm
	Dinner #2 Time	7:15pm
	Potty Patrol Check	Brown, Solid, Normal (7:30pm)
NIGHT	Night Vitamins & Supplements	(usual + cal) 9:00pm without food
	Bedtime Snack (optional)	10:00pm
BEFORE BED	Bedtime Med Time	9:45pm
	Potty Patrol Check	None
	Other Notes	
		Slept all night in bed
		No barking during the day
		No vomiting in the morning
		Ate Chicken, Veg., Pasta Stew
		Added Calcium to Night Vitamins

Since I am still improving Norman's diet, I often run across something else that Norman cannot tolerate. I use the same approach when trying new items and to determine what is causing gas, stomach and gastrointestinal problems. I have found that, when liver disease is present, gastrointestinal problems frequently occur when something new is not tolerated in the diet.

Soon after this crisis, I received a call from the person who would become Norman's veterinarian. I had found a list of Holistic Vet's on the Internet and e-mailed one that was in my area. I had called during the crisis and she got back to me after it was over. When she called, I was pretty hard on her. I asked her a lot of questions and explained Norman's history briefly. I told her I was looking for a Vet who would take other alternative treatments into consideration and work with me on Norman's diet and supplements to help me take the best possible care of him. Dr. Forster answered all my questions and we scheduled a visit for her to come over to my house and take a fresh look at Norman's case. In order to do this, I needed to get all of Norman's Vet records from his previous Vet. Dr. Forster gave me great insight into what all the blood test results meant and the sonogram diagnosis. This fresh look at Norman's history was very educational and enlightening for me.

Notes on Blood Test Results

Blood test results should be used to look at the BIG picture. Never take one value by itself. Although some are very specific to liver disease, they should be looked at in relation to all other values. Also, keep in mind that blood test numbers are specific to the machine used to perform the test and should not be compared. Instead, compare the results to the reference range. "Flagging ranges" identify results that are out of the reference range and are usually printed in bold. Flagging ranges are just a guide. Consult your Vet for specific medical interpretations.

Liver Specific blood tests:

ALT – is a liver-specific leakage enzyme that is high when the body is losing cells.
AST – occurs in the liver, determined in conjunction with other liver tests (ALT, GGT).
Bilirubin – is formed in the liver before excretion in the bile.
Cholesterol – is produced in the liver and synthesized into bile acids. Low levels may indicate liver disease.
GGT – is an enzyme originating from the liver and is used in conjunction with other liver tests.
Potassium – low levels may indicate chronic liver disease.

Find the Cause, don't just Treat the Symptoms.

One of the most important first steps in treating liver disease is finding the cause. Without knowing the source of the problem, you are only treating the symptoms. Dr. Forster's initial consultation and review of Norman's history not only helped me understand his condition, it also identified several red flags. Those red flags were then looked at with 20/20 hind-sight (perfect vision) and used to determine the best course of treatment.

Review of History reveals Red Flags.

The first major red flag was that 3 months before Norman was diagnosed with liver disease, I had taken him in to have his teeth cleaned and annual vaccinations. The blood test done before the teeth cleaning showed that his test for liver disease (ALT) was normal, but he was Anemic (low red blood cell count).

During and after this visit, Norman's body was bombarded with drugs and chemicals.

- He was injected with pain medication to remove a small growth on his ear.
- He was given anesthesia for the dental cleaning.
- He was given all of his vaccinations (Rabies, DHLP/Parvo).
- He was given antibiotics for 20 days after the cleaning.
- He continued taking Rimadyl for Arthritis pain.
- He continued taking monthly Heartgard tablets to guard against heartworms.
- He continued taking monthly Flea & Tick control medication.

If Norman's liver was already damaged, all of this medication pushed him over the edge. The Anemia could have been a sign that he was not in the best condition to have all of this done at once.

The next red flag was his Gingivitis. Bad teeth and gums produce toxins that are harmful to the liver. And, it's a general sign of bad health.

Finally, I couldn't help but kick myself for giving him NSAID pain killers (Rimadyl) for his Osteoarthritis on a daily basis for over 2 years.

This reminded me of his not-so-severe symptoms of loose stools, constant drooling and gas, which I had ignored for years.

Of course, I was also feeding him the expensive commercial pet food (with rice). I had taken him in for gas and a sensitive stomach 7-years ago and never even considered that the pet food was the problem. I had been taught to feed Norman "the good pet food" and thought I was giving him the very best available.

I Didn't Know!

I feel like I didn't know anything before all of this happened. I didn't know to ask questions. I didn't know medications could have harmful side effects. I didn't know commercial pet-food could contain toxins. I didn't know bad breath, drooling and gas were signs of poor health.

Well, now I know. So, I question everything now, and I do my research. I'm educating myself and, hopefully, educating other well-meaning dog-lovers to do the same.

My Conclusions

I can't say for sure what caused Norman's liver disease. But, I've come to the conclusion that it was probably caused by a combination of: long-term use of NSAID pain killers, untreated Gingivitis, food sensitivities (rice), over vaccinating, old-age, and poor diet (not-so-healthy commercial pet food), combined with a dog breed that has a tendency to have liver problems.

Now that we knew what caused the liver disease, Dr. Forster helped me formulate the best treatment for Norman.

Dr. Forster's Prescribed Supplements and Vitamins.

Dr. Forster then did her own research and consulted another Holistic Vet and an Internist to give me additional information. She recommended other supplements and vitamins.

- Taurine 500mg 2x/day (for both liver and cognitive)
- L-Carnitine 500mg 2x/day (for both liver and cognitive)
- Alpha-Lipoic acid (ala) 100mg 1x/day (for cognitive)

- Vitamin E 200 mg + general antioxidant formula d alpha form not dl alpha
- Double dose of Milk Thistle (from150mg a day to 150mg 2x/day)
- Add Turmeric (spice) (1 tsp daily) to his food – start small at first
- Canine Plus Multi-Vitamin with antioxidants from Vetri-Science (available from your Vet)
- Prozyme Digestive Enzymes instead of other brand (available from your Vet)

Notes on Supplements and Vitamins: I list brand names along with contents when available so that you can find your own source of these supplements and vitamins. There is a lot of variability in different brands, and sometimes they may not actually contain what is claimed on the label. So, stick with well-known and proven brands. I am not advertising for these items, only for their effectiveness in treating liver disease.

A complete list with recommended dosages has been compiled for your use (see Appendix A).

Since I started feeding Norman homemade dog food, specialized for his liver disease and added the additional supplements and vitamins, he has been sick four times. These were related to diet or arthritis. Each time he got sick I learned something new about how his diet (intake) affects his system.

Trial and Error – Adjusting Diet to Norman's Needs

I wish I could tell you that developing the perfect diet for Norman was easy, and that I got it right the first time. But, that's just not the way it happened.

Instead, I would develop a meal, let Norman eat it for several days or weeks and watch to see how he did on it. Sometimes the meal would be great for a few days, and then he'd be sick again. I'd go back to the drawing board to find out what went wrong and try again.

- I've gone from preparing each meal from scratch using strictly all "natural" ingredients to canned food from a Health Food Store, and everything in between.
- I've been an extremist where I made each meal using fresh vegetables and soy protein.
- I've been economical where I made large batches of cooked food and froze it for use over several weeks.
- I've been lazy and used healthy canned food.
- I've used hot water to heat his food, and I've used the microwave to heat his food.
- I've used raw beef, turkey, liver and bones, cooked chicken, beef and liver, tofu, soy granules, yogurt, cottage cheese, potatoes, yams, pasta, couscous, millet, barley, oatmeal, fresh fruit, dried fruit, fresh vegetables, frozen vegetables, and canned vegetables.
- I've tried healthy commercial food like Halo Canned Food and Sojo grain mixes that go with raw meat.

I don't know if I can say, "I've tried it all." But I've definitely tried many different recipes over the last year. And, I've learned a lot along the way.

Now you have the benefit of learning my lessons without having to go through it yourself.

The rest of this book is the compilation and presentation of all my research. The goal is that you will be able to digest this information quickly, and start putting together your own homemade diet with supplements for your dog. As I found out with Norman, there is no "perfect diet" for all dogs. That is the main reason the prescription diet for liver disease did not work for him. It is a one-size-fits-all recipe. You will need to do your own experiments with the ingredients and recipes that I give you to find what works for your dog. I recommend that you also work with a good Vet who believes in the use of homemade diets and natural supplements.

Over a year and a half after Norman's initial diagnosis, he is doing great. The last blood test a month ago came back with everything still normal. (See Appendix C for a complete history of test results)

Final Note – Treating Pain Associated with Arthritis

Norman also has Arthritis in his hips and knees. This is why he was on pain medication for so long. Now that he has a damaged liver, he can't have any of the typical pain medications.

About nine months after I started Norman on a healthy diet and supplements for liver disease, he gave me a scare. Norman had been a ravenous eater and very excited around mealtime. But now he was more than just excited. He was anxious, restless, drooling, panting, crying (barking), not sleeping for more than 2 hours at a time, inhaling his food, pacing around the house, hunting for cat poop outside, and eating it.

I tried everything. I tried various homeopathic remedies for gastritis. I changed his diet, increasing and decreasing the amount of protein and fat in his food. I gave him more Vitamin C and B12. I gave him Bach's Rescue Remedy. I fasted him for a day. I gave him Gas-X. Nothing worked.

After 5 days of trying everything I knew to try, I took him in to see Dr. Forster. We did blood tests and everything was still normal. Her guess was that he was in pain. But we didn't know why. We decided to try a pain medication called Torbutrol.

I gave him the medication and fed him as usual. I left him alone for a couple of hours and when I returned he had urinated and soiled the house. He was lying on the floor as if he couldn't get up. His mouth was dripping wet from panting constantly. His back legs were so weak he could barely stand to potty. He was limping on his back left leg. He was so restless he wouldn't sit or lie down. He just kept walking around or standing with his head in a corner.

I called Dr. Forster and described his condition. She offered to come over (at 9:30pm) but said, even if she did, there wasn't anything she could do until morning at the clinic. She didn't think it was life threatening, but I had never seen him act this upset before. I was a scared, frantic mother afraid this was going to be the end for Norman. The best thing she told me was to get control of my emotions because my emotional state was affecting Norman.

She was right. I was an emotional basket case! I was so worried he was going to die I worked myself up into a panic. I immediately prayed for peace and for Norman's health.

Norman and I finally went to bed, but it was the longest night of my life. Norman got up every couple of hours, and I got up with him. Finally, at 7:30am we went to see Dr. Forster at the clinic. She worked Norman and me in as soon as possible. He was still acting the same. She said he looked like he was in pain. She kept him at the clinic to do x-rays and other tests to figure out what was causing the pain.

I left him there and went off to take care of myself. When she had the test results back, she called me to tell me why he was in so much pain. His back hip has severe Osteoarthritis, irregular joint surface and severely calcified discs. At his age and condition, surgery was not an option. She recommended that I try acupuncture for the pain.

I took Norman for six acupuncture treatments but, ultimately, I found diet change and homeopathic remedies for arthritis and pain worked best to keep the pain under control.

Without homeopathic remedies for arthritis pain, I would have had to put Norman to sleep. He was in a lot of pain. But now, he is doing fine. He still has a limp. But he has no signs of anxiety, crying (barking), restlessness or panting. He sleeps throughout the night, sleeps most of the day and seems to be comfortable. He doesn't hunt for cat poop anymore and waits patiently to be fed.

It WORKS!

I am convinced that alternative treatments for liver disease and arthritis in the form of diet, supplements and homeopathic medications WORK. I wouldn't be writing this book if they didn't. I know that I would NOT have Norman with me today if they didn't work. I wouldn't be recommending them to you if I didn't believe with all my heart they are safe as well as good for your dog.

I hope you find the answers you're looking for, or at least the hope to keep looking for a way to help your dog heal. I know that if you love your dog as much as I love Norman that you will want to know everything you can do to keep him at your side for as long as your dog isn't suffering.

I pray that you have as much success with your homemade healthy dog food and supplements as I have. I encourage you to ask your Veterinarian questions. Don't give up without trying. And, take good care of yourself and your dog. You'll feel better knowing you did everything you could for your dog.

Chapter 2 – Liver Disease & Cirrhosis

"If you do not hope, you will not find what is beyond your hopes." – St. Clement

Liver disease and Cirrhosis are difficult to explain. This is my basic understanding of the disease, but it is far from complete. I gleaned this information from several sources. It is important for you to have a basic knowledge of what liver disease is, so you understand how it will affect your dog, and so that you can better care for your dog.

Liver Disease -- What is it?

Liver disease is the fifth leading cause of non-accidental death among dogs. It is a very serious condition. Since the liver is the largest and most important organ in the body, the body becomes toxic and starts to deteriorate if it's not working properly.

The liver is a complex organ. It filters your dog's entire blood supply many times each day. It processes everything that the body is exposed to, both internally and externally. It performs many vital functions, including detoxifying the blood of drugs and poisons; removing ammonia and other wastes from the blood; manufacturing blood-clotting factors; and synthesizing enzymes, proteins and metabolites.

The liver has a phenomenal ability to regain function and is believed to be capable of complete regeneration. When liver disease is identified early on, there is a chance of complete recovery. However, early diagnosis and treatment of liver disease is extremely difficult. The liver can perform its function without discernible changes in blood analyses with up to 75 percent of it affected by disease. This means the disease is usually well advanced, and possibly untreatable, before any symptoms are noted.

Liver disease is a catch-all term that applies to any medical disorder that affects the liver. There are many different specific and non-specific diseases of the liver. Your Vet will need to do further diagnosis to

19

determine the cause and best treatment. Because of the complexity of liver disease, I am going to cover it using a very abbreviated bullet format. I will keep the rest of this chapter as simple as possible, sticking to the most important points.

Liver Disease -- Diagnosis

Here is what you can expect your Vet to do in order to diagnose your dog's specific form of liver disease.

- Examination – to identify the specific signs of liver disease.
- Consultation with Vet – (most important) to get a full history (when, where, why, how, etc.) and more to determine when the liver disease started and what could be causing it, so that whatever's causing it can be stopped.
- Blood Test – to check for anemia, other organic abnormalities, health of the bile system, infections, electrolyte imbalances, digestive enzymes, blood parasites, blood proteins, blood sugar (glucose), liver enzymes and ammonia.
- Pre- and Post-Meal Bile Acid Test – to compare the two blood levels (pre and post meal) allows the veterinarian to see how well the liver, bile ducts, and blood flow to the liver are functioning. Bile acids are removed from liver (portal) blood by the liver cells. If the liver cells are not functioning well, the bile acids remain in circulation and enter the body (systemic) blood supply where they are measured by this test.
- Ultrasound – to visually inspect for scar tissue, cancer, abscesses, abnormal blood supply, to determine what percentage of the liver is affected and determine the size and density of the liver, gall bladder and bile system.
- Biopsy – to give a microscopic perspective to ascertain diagnosis, the actual conditions of the liver cells and prognosis to better determine appropriate treatment.

Liver Disease -- Treatments

There is a wide range of treatments for the various liver diseases. Your Vet will be able to recommend the best treatment. Here are the basic points for treatment of liver disease.

Conventional Treatment

- There are no conventional medications that actually cure liver disease.
- Identify and remove all toxic drugs or agents, which may potentially hurt the liver.
- Rest and confinement to allow the body time to heal the liver, reduce discomfort, and reduce physical and mental stress.
- Change diet to "get down to basics" and provide all necessary nutrients, which may be lost due to liver processing failure, being careful not to over-tax the liver with large amounts of food. (Usually done with a prescription diet dog food.)
- Control ascites and water retention with reduced sodium.
- Control concurrent infections with antibiotics.
- Add Vitamin and Mineral supplement.
- Deal with other medical problems as they come up. Deal with each separate problem both individually and as part of the whole diseased entity with regular trips to the Vet.

Alternative Treatment

- Discuss nutritional needs and supplements with your Vet before changing the diet and adding supplements to make sure you are doing no harm (e.g. high protein with concurrent kidney problems could cause kidney failure).
- Change to natural or healthy homemade diet with high levels of top quality protein, which will not produce high levels of ammonia during digestion, and high levels of carbohydrates with at least 6% of essential fatty acids.
- Adjust diet to add food remedies that support liver function.
- Add Milk Thistle, Vitamin E, Selenium, SAM-e and other supplements that support liver function (as recommended by your Vet).
- Add a high quality multi-vitamin with minerals and anti-oxidants.
- Add digestive enzymes to meals to aid in utilization of food and supplements.
- Remove all toxic chemicals from the environment, including the diet, pesticides, chemical treatments and medications.
- Treat the whole system, including new problems as they come

up.
- Perform regular checkups at home and see your Vet regularly to monitor progress and check blood levels.

Liver Disease -- Causes

- Prolonged use of some drugs such as NSAID's (Non-Steroidal Anti-Inflammatory Drug), cortisone, anti-convulsants, steroids, some antibiotics, anesthetics, parasite control drugs, chemotherapy drugs and acetaminophen.
- Exposure to high levels of toxic chemicals like insecticides, lead, phosphorus, selenium, arsenic and iron.
- Other diseases, viruses and infections like hepatitis, heartworms, infections elsewhere in the body; most commonly dental disease, chronic skin and ear infections.
- Certain breeds of dogs are prone to genetically inherited liver disease (female Doberman Pinschers, American and English Cocker Spaniels, Bedlington Terriers, West Highland White Terriers).
- In-breeding.

Liver Disease -- Common Symptoms

- Vomiting with or without blood.
- Diarrhea with or without blood.
- Eating unusual things.
- Frequent urination and increased water intake.
- Depression or lethargy – doesn't want to play anymore, lays in a spot away from you and family.
- Loss of appetite or ravenous appetite.
- Orange urine.
- Pale gray stools or orange/yellow stools.
- Jaundice – the whites of the eyes, skin and gums turn yellow.
- Chronic weight loss or wasting.
- Ascites - swollen belly filled with fluid.
- Severe neurological signs - behavioral changes, seizures, aimless pacing or circling, head pressing. (May be associated with mealtime.)
- Unexplained bleeding or prolonged bleeding (e.g. after nail trimming or drawing blood).

Cirrhosis of the Liver

Cirrhosis is the final stage of liver disease. It is when the liver cells die off and turn into scar tissue. This condition is irreversible. The only treatment option is dietary care. The liver can still function with up to 70-80 percent of the liver affected. Cellular regeneration is not possible once the tissue is scarred. The only hope is to keep the part of the liver that remains as healthy as possible.

Chapter 3 – Healthy Homemade Dog Food for Liver Disease

"Let food be thy medicine." – Hippocrates

Healthy Dog Food Basics

A healthy diet is the cornerstone for treating canine liver disease. This section covers the basic food groups in the Healthy Homemade Dog Food Recipes and how they should be used, or not used, in the treatment of liver disease.

Food Groups
Protein

Proteins must be of high biological quality to reduce the production of ammonia, which is a by-product of protein digestion. Normal amounts of protein should be fed to your dog unless your Vet recommends protein restriction. The liver needs protein during repair. Red meat and eggs tend to produce high levels of ammonia, which is toxic to the liver. Milk or soy-based proteins like cottage cheese, yogurt and tofu are the best.

Meat

Raw meat is usually the recommended source of natural protein for a dog. Most natural diets are made up of raw beef, chicken and turkey muscle and organ meat. However, dogs with liver disease need an alternative protein source.

Caution: Raw meat can be contaminated. If you do decide to use raw meat, mix 4 drops of Grape seed extract and distilled water with the meat to kill the bacteria. If switching to raw meat, start small and increase gradually.

Natural Health Bible for Dogs & Cats reports: "Studies show that dogs with liver disease fed diets containing meat-based proteins have shorter survival times and more severe clinical signs than dogs with liver disease fed milk-based or soy-based protein diets."

For this reason, **raw meat is not recommended**. If your dog will not eat milk-based or soy-based protein, then another alternative is to feed high quality cooked (boiled) muscle and organ meat. These include chicken, ground turkey or high quality ground beef. Only serve one type of meat at a time (e.g. do not mix beef with turkey).

Soy
Soy protein is preferred over raw meat to decrease the formation of chemicals that may be toxic to your dog. Soy protein is growing in popularity with people, which makes it easier to find for your dog. The most common soy-based source of protein is tofu. You can also use soy granules, which are cheaper than tofu and easier to store and serve.

Fish
Cod fillets or white low-fat fish has a specific amino acid that actually helps heal the liver. Soy and fat-free cottage cheese also have this specific amino acid.

Dairy Products
Milk-based products are usually not needed in a natural diet. However, yogurt and cottage cheese are high quality sources of protein, which do not produce high levels of ammonia during digestion. Always use the fat-free natural or plain forms. **Watch out for lactose intolerance!** If your dog has diarrhea after eating a meal with a milk-based product, that's a good sign that he's lactose intolerant and you should omit milk products from the diet.

Eggs
Eggs are another source of protein but, like meat, they are not as good as soy. If you use eggs as a source of protein, be sure to use eggs that come from free-roaming nesting hens. Raw eggs can contain bacteria, so it is best to serve your dog soft-boiled or lightly scrambled eggs.

Carbohydrates

High levels of high quality, highly digestible carbohydrates are needed to supply energy. Carbohydrates like pasta and potatoes are recommended. Vegetables are a good source of complex carbohydrates and help remove intestinal toxins from the body.

Grains

Grains are not found in the true natural diet, but some people add them for nutritional value. Grains must be cooked to be digested. Most dogs usually accept quick-cooking and economical grains such as oatmeal and rice. However, grains do break down into sugars and can cause yeast overgrowth. Since grains are so high in glucose, they bombard the liver. Grains, like milk-based products, are mucus-forming (toxic fungal growth) and may contribute to health problems such as allergies, ear infections, skin problems, bloating, joint problems, malabsorption and digestive disorders.

For this reason, **grains are not recommended** for regular use in your dog's diet. Then, only freshly cooked grains that have nutritional or healing value are recommended at all. Do not serve cooked grains that have been refrigerated for more than 1 day. The fermentation is harmful to the liver.

Pasta and Potatoes Instead of Grains

Instead of using grains, pasta and potatoes are the best source of carbohydrates. Like grains, pasta and potatoes provide energy in the form of calories. They have the added benefit of stopping heartburn by absorbing acid in the stomach. Pasta and potatoes do not ferment, so they won't cause digestive problems like grains.

Pasta can be cooked separately or with vegetables. To get the most out of potatoes, wash and cook with the peel. The best way to cook potatoes is in the microwave. It helps retain the nutrients that are lost when boiling in water. Potatoes have been listed as foods to avoid in some books. They are listed under the same category as the deadly nightshade plants and thought to be toxic. But, botanists have proven that potatoes are actually very safe for humans and your dog. If your potatoes have eyes that are green, remove them. The stems, leaves, eyes and flowers of potato plants are toxic and dangerous.

Vegetables

Vegetables are usually only a small part of a natural diet, used to add vitamins, minerals and roughage to the diet. However, many vegetables have healing properties for the liver and play a key role in the diet. **It is best to use a variety of vegetables and rotate their use**. Do not use the same ones repeatedly, and do not give too many at one time. Some vegetables like beets and garlic should only be used in small quantities. Others, like onions, should be avoided all together.

To aid in digestion, some should be cooked. Others can be served raw as long as they are chopped or pulped in a form that is easily digestible. Serving suggestions are given for each vegetable. The most important thing to remember about serving vegetables is – **variety**. A list of vegetable combinations and substitutions are given with the recipes. You can use fresh or frozen, organic or non-organic. Be sure to wash all fresh produce thoroughly to remove residual insecticides, dyes and waxes.

Bones

Raw bones in a Natural Diet are like candy to a dog. Dogs love to eat them, and some do a good job of digesting them. However, they are **not recommended** for use in your dog's diet for liver disease, because some dogs will have intestinal, digestive difficulties. Some of these difficulties could be fatal, or at least require surgery to get through it. Surgery or additional health problems are too great a risk for dogs with liver disease. These health risks outweigh the benefits of bones.

To ensure your dog is getting enough bone minerals – give a human grade bonemeal supplement or bonemeal tablets. For cleaning teeth – there are tooth brushes and gel rinses. For jaw exercise, massaging gums and relieving stress – use safe chew toys.

Seeds and Nuts

Seeds and nuts are a good source of protein and fat. They are best digested when fresh, raw and unsalted, as a nut-butter or finely ground. Nuts are a great addition to the soy-based diet. They add the needed fat that is hard to get. Use small amounts of sliced almonds, pumpkin seeds and flax seeds. They are also a good source of Omega-3 and Omega-6 fatty acids.

Oil
Vegetable oils like extra virgin olive oil are excellent sources of linoleic acid and important unsaturated fatty acids that dogs need. Use cold-pressed safflower, soy, olive or corn oil.

Fruit
Fruits are good for the occasional treat or snack. Many dogs like dried fruits such as figs, dates, prunes and apricots as well as fresh fruits like bananas, apples and berries. Fruits are a good source of vitamins and minerals, especially potassium. For easy digestion, feed fruit as an in-between treat or snack at least 1 hour before or after a regular meal. Do not feed your dog citrus fruit (e.g. oranges, grapefruit, tangerines).

Spices
Some common flavorings used in a natural diet are garlic and nutritional yeast. These add flavor and have some benefits. However, nutritional yeast can cause allergies or digestive problems in some dogs. Fresh garlic is beneficial for toning up the digestive track and preventing fleas and worms. Some other spices that are healing for the liver and digestive tract are dried basil leaves and turmeric. Use these gradually in all of your dog's meals.

Water

Give your dog distilled water for the first month. Distilled water is free of dissolved minerals and, because of this, has the special property of being able to actively absorb toxic substances from the body and eliminate them. Studies validate the benefits of drinking distilled water when cleansing or detoxifying the system for short periods of time. Do not cook with distilled water or give your dog distilled water during a fast.

Spring water or water filtered through reverse osmosis are acceptable for regular use. Always keep fresh water available for your dog in a ceramic, stainless steel or lead-free glass dish. Never use plastic dishes for food or water bowls. Some of the recipes will use water to mix with the food. When there is water in a meal, your dog will drink less water from his bowl. This is normal and should not cause alarm.

How Much to Feed in How Many Servings

Most Natural Diets tell you to feed your dog as much as he will eat in 1 or 2 servings while watching his weight. This works for healthy dogs that aren't lethargic, ravenous, pot-bellied or losing weight. But for the dog with liver disease, volume and number of servings is important. It's important not to let your dog go without eating enough to sustain himself, and not to let your dog eat so much that it overloads his liver.

Depending on the type of liver disease you may need to decrease the amount of protein. Discuss your dog's specific diet needs with your Vet.

To be as easy on the liver as possible, meals should be broken down into small portions and fed more frequently than a normal diet. Serve your dog 3-4 small meals a day along with a small nighttime fruit snack (if needed).

Why Diet and Supplements Work for Liver Disease

There is nothing magical about this treatment. It works because of the liver's ability to regenerate, and it is the liver that processes the food and supplements.

"Dietary therapy is a mainstay of treating the dog with liver disease, as there are few conventional medications that actually treat liver disease."
- *Natural Health Bible for Dogs & Cats*

A healthy diet for liver disease includes:

- High quality and highly digestible carbohydrates for energy.
- Frequent feedings of high quality carbohydrates, such as pasta and potatoes, are recommended.
- Vegetables provide complex carbohydrates, fiber and vitamins

to remove toxins.

- High biological valued protein to reduce the production of ammonia.
- Digestive enzymes to help the liver process and digest the food.
- Multi-Vitamin and Supplements to balance nutritional needs.
- Pure drinking water (for drinking and in all recipes).

What's Wrong with Commercial Foods or Prescription Foods?

Here are the basic reasons for not using commercial pet foods:

- Commercial pet foods use low quality protein sources (such as meat and bonemeal that are easily contaminated with bacteria) that are cooked to kill bacteria. However cooking cannot kill a bacterial by-product (endotoxins). Nothing can be done to remove endotoxins from contaminated pet food. Endotoxins can cause illness in dogs.
- Commercial pet foods contain raw grain products like peanut and cottonseed meal. Toxins from mold (common in raw grains) may also contaminate and cause illness.
- Commercial pet foods use poor quality ingredients that most people couldn't eat.
- Nutritional needs vary for each pet, and commercial foods do not provide for the individual and specific nutritional needs.

Homemade Dog Food is the Only Way to Go

There's no question that the freshest, most wholesome diet, over which you have the most control, is a homemade diet. Only by preparing your dog's food at home can you exercise complete control over the quality and the type of ingredients that your dog will eat. A homemade diet allows you to easily adjust nutrient levels as well as composition to meet your dog's changing needs.

"For dogs with various medical problems ... a homemade diet is probably the best way to go, as no 'natural' prepared diets at this time serve the needs of pets with medical disorders. There are medical-type 'prescription' diets for dogs with various diseases, but these do not always contain [appropriate] ingredients [for liver disease] and may contain by-products and chemicals not desired by owners who opt for holistic care for their pets." (*Natural Health Bible for Dogs & Cats*) (Author's additions in brackets.)

Creating a balanced diet is actually quite simple and only requires a few supplements. The optimum amount of any specific nutrient is not always well known. You should work with your Vet to determine your dog's specific nutritional needs.

How to Prepare a Homemade Meal
Food Preparation Guidelines
When preparing your homemade meals, it's best to keep your food groups in separate containers. In case one spoils, you will not lose everything. Then at mealtime, all you have to do is combine all the ingredients, along with any medicine and enzymes, then serve.

It's best to only prepare enough food for a few days at a time if you store the food in your refrigerator. You don't want to take any chances of giving your dog rancid or spoiled food. If you have extra storage space in your freezer, you can prepare more food, freeze it and use as needed.

Preparing Meat
- Buy 1-3 pounds of high quality meat, like skinless, boneless chicken parts (thighs, or breasts) or a young hen. If buying in bulk, separate into 3 days worth of servings, wrap in plastic wrap and freeze in a freezer bag. 3-day servings range from 1 - 3 pieces of chicken.
- Take out one 3-day serving of chicken from the freezer and place in the refrigerator to thaw overnight.
- Bring the chicken to a boil in 2-4 cups of water and cook on medium for 5-10 minutes while skimming the fat off the top. Once the fat is cooked off the chicken, add optional spices like basil, garlic and kelp, then simmer on low for 45 minutes to an hour. Turn heat off and allow time to cool. Remove any bones, and chop into bite size pieces.
- Refrigerate with broth in a food storage container for up to 3 days.

- Freeze what cannot be consumed in 3 days to use later.

Preparing Liver or Other Organ Meat

- Buy 1 pound of chicken liver and separate into individual servings by cutting the liver into bite-size pieces. Put the pieces in a small container or freezer bag. Individual servings range from 1 Tbsp – ½ pound.
- Take out 1-3 servings of meat from the freezer and place in the refrigerator to thaw overnight.
- Bring the meat to a boil in 2-4 cups of water and cook on medium for 5-10 minutes while skimming the fat off the top. Once the fat is cooked off the raw meat, add optional spices like basil, garlic, and kelp, then simmer on low for 20 - 30 minutes. Turn heat off and allow time to cool.
- Refrigerate with broth in a food storage container for up to 3 days.
- Freeze what cannot be consumed in 3 days to use later.

Preparing Fresh Vegetables

- Buy 3 fresh vegetables at a time (e.g. 1 bunch of carrots, 3 stalks of broccoli, and 2 stalks of celery).
- Wash 3-9 servings of three different raw vegetables (e.g. carrots, broccoli, celery). One serving of each vegetable ranges from 1 to 4 tablespoons. Combined daily servings of vegetables range from ¼ to 1 cup.
- Chop the vegetables with a knife, food processor, grater or blender. For small dogs you want them extremely fine. Medium-size dogs need coarsely chopped, and large dogs need small bite-size pieces.
- Lightly steam (1-3 minutes) vegetables like carrots, broccoli and cauliflower to help with digestion.
- Combine and refrigerate in a food storage container for up to 3 days.

Preparing Frozen Vegetables

- Cook 3-9 servings of frozen vegetables as directed on package. Daily servings of frozen vegetables range from ¼ to 1 cup.
- For small dogs, chop the cooked vegetables in a food processor or blender.
- Refrigerate separately in a food storage container for up to 3 days.

Preparing Grains, Potatoes, Yams, and Other Items

- **Grains** – Cook 3-6 servings as directed on the package. Daily servings of grains range from ¼ to 1 cup. Refrigerate separately in a food storage container for up to 1 day.
- **Pasta** – Cook 3-9 servings as directed on the package. Daily servings of cooked pasta range from ¼ to 1 cup. 1 cup of uncooked pasta yields roughly 4 cups of cooked pasta. Refrigerate separately in a food storage container for up to 3 days.
- **Potatoes/Yams** – Bake or microwave 2-6 medium sized potatoes at a time. Daily servings of potatoes range from ¼ to 1 ½ potatoes/yams. Refrigerate separately in a food storage container for up to 3 days.
- **Eggs** – Soft-boil (5-15 minutes) 1-6 large free-range eggs at a time. Daily servings of eggs range from 1 to 6 eggs. Refrigerate unpeeled for up to 1 week.
- **Fish** – Poach fillet in a frying pan with water until fish is white. Daily servings of fish range from ¼ to 1 cup. Refrigerate for up to 2 days.
- **Broth** – Bring 1 small chicken or 1 pound of beef neck bones (about 4 bones) to boil in 2-4 quarts of water for 5-10 minutes while skimming the fat off the top. Once the fat is cooked off, simmer on low for 1 hour or until completely cooked. Allow broth to cool, then remove the bones and freeze in small to medium size containers until needed. Be sure to leave room in the container for the broth to expand as it freezes. Thaw in the refrigerator the night before and use within 1 week.

Foods That Heal

This table of food items shows what that food item contains and the function or benefit of that food item in general and in relation to liver disease.

Food Item	Contains	Benefits
Artichokes	Silymarin, Folate and Vitamin C	Helps prevent cancer and heal liver damage.
Alfalfa Sprouts	Vitamin K	Build healthy digestive track and prevent bleeding.
Soy Beans	Amino acids, L-Arginine	Help detoxify ammonia, a byproduct of protein digestion.
Kidney Beans	Amino acids, L-Arginine	Help detoxify ammonia, a byproduct of protein digestion.
Peas	Amino acids, L-Arginine	Help detoxify ammonia, a byproduct of protein digestion.
Seeds (flax, pumpkin, etc...)	Amino acids, L-Arginine	Help detoxify ammonia, a byproduct of protein digestion.
Parsley	Myristicin, Apiol, Vitamin C	Help pass more urine to remove infection in urinary tract and help digestion.
Beets	Vitamin B, Iron, Beta-carotene	An antioxidant that protects against cancer.
Carrots	Beta-carotene, Vitamin A	An antioxidant that fights free radicals.
Raisins	Potassium	Help keep digestion and blood healthy.
Pineapple	Bromine	Helps treat all liver conditions, aids digestion and helps joint function.
Kelp	Folate, Vitamin B, Magnesium, Vitamin C.	Small amounts are beneficial for the heart and blood.
Blueberries	Vitamin C, Leukotrenes	Prevent cancer and constipation. Reduce risk of infection.
Raspberries	Vitamin C, Leukotrenes	Prevent cancer and constipation. Reduce risk of infection.
Cranberries	Vitamin C, Leukotrenes	Prevent cancer and constipation. Reduce risk of infection.

Food Item	Contains	Benefits
Blackberries	Vitamin C, Leukotrenes	Prevent cancer and constipation. Reduce risk of infection.
Garlic	Selenium	Reduce risk of stomach and colon cancer. Ease digestive upset and reduce gas.
Barley	Vitamin E, Selenium	Improve digestion, protect against cancer, reduce blood clots.
Basil	Unknown beneficial substances.	Ease digestive disorders, protect against cancer.
Turmeric	Phytochemicals (or Phytonutrients), Curcumin	Antioxidant that prevents colon cancer, anti-inflammatory for arthritis, decreases gas formation and spasms, prevent stomach ulcers.
Apples	Quercetin, Insoluble fiber and Soluble fiber called Pectin	Prevent cancer and prevent or relieve constipation. Reduce cholesterol produced in the liver. Slows digestion.
Potatoes	Anticarcinogenic Chlorogenic acid, Potassium, Vitamin C, Folate	Help prevent cancer and control high blood pressure.
Sweet Potato	Beta-carotene, Vitamins C & E	Preserve memory. Prevent cancer and heart disease.
Prunes	Insoluble and Soluble fiber, Sorbitol, Beta-carotene, and Potassium.	Relieve constipation. Lower cholesterol. Reduce risk of cancer and heart disease.
Squash	Rich array of Vitamins, Minerals and Nutrients like Vitamin C and Beta-carotene	Help prevent cancer and lung problems.
Broccoli	Beta-carotene, Sulforaphane, I3C, Vitamin C, Folate, Calcium and Fiber.	Fight off cancer, boost immunity and protect against heart disease.
Celery	Insoluble fiber, Potassium, Vitamin C and Calcium.	Reduce high blood pressure and lower the risk of cancer.

Health Fact
Garlic is a powerful detoxifying agent that can protect against various liver toxins.

Healthy Treats

If you're like most dog owners, giving your dog a treat is a regular part of your routine. Now, you can replace those dog bone treats from the store with these healthy treats that actually help your dog heal.

Fruit is a great treat and can be given often. As a guideline, give only a few pieces of these listed fruit items at a time. Don't over do it. Avoid giving citrus fruit of any kind, and give fruit treats at least an hour after meals or before bed.

- Prunes
- Blueberries
- Raspberries
- Bananas
- Cranberries
- Blackberries
- Pineapple chunks (used sparingly due to high acidity)

Chapter 4 – Healthy Homemade Dog Food Recipes

"It is not easy to be a pioneer – but oh, it is fascinating! I wouldn't trade one moment, even the worst moment, for all the riches in the world." – Elizabeth Blackwell

Here are some recipes I have worked with over the last year. They are a good place to start.

Tip: Use Ziploc® bags or the new Microwave/Freezer safe storage containers (like Glad®) to store and freeze extra portions when you make a recipe. Thaw each container for at least 24 hours in the refrigerator. Or, defrost in the microwave in microwave safe container.

Sunny's Miracle Diet

By: Kennalea Pratt

This recipe gave me hope. This includes the supplements and a Healthy Powder used in the diet. It includes brown rice, which is hard to digest, and oatmeal, which can ferment easily. This shows you where I started and what inspired me. Many "liver dogs" have done very well on this diet.

3	Pounds of ground turkey
4	Cups brown rice
¼	Teaspoon garlic powder
11	Cups (or more) water
1	Bag frozen mixed vegetables
1	Bag frozen chopped broccoli
1	Cup regular oatmeal

1. Combine water, turkey and rice in a large stew pot and bring to a boil, cover and reduce heat to low and cook for 45 min.
2. Add 1 bag of mixed vegetables.
3. Add 1 bag of chopped broccoli.
4. Stir in thoroughly, cover and cook for about 5 minutes.
5. Stir in 1 cup (¼ cup at a time) of regular oatmeal until all water is absorbed.
6. Put one lukewarm serving in food bowl.
7. Add ½ tablespoon of Modified Healthy Powder, 5 drops of Teeter Creeks LVR-TONE, 5 drops of Milk Thistle Extract and ½ digestive enzyme capsule into meal and serve.

Meat substitutes:
You can substitute the highest-grade ground beef for the ground turkey.

Meal variations:
Add 1 chopped boiled egg to meal. Mix ¼ cup of non-fat cottage cheese with the meal.

Reheat:
Put serving in microwave safe bowl and heat for 1 minute or just long enough to reach room temperature.

Store the unused food in containers and refrigerate enough for 3 days. Freeze the rest.

Yield: *About 22 cups.*

Serving suggestions (in cups):
small dog – ¾ to 1¾; medium – 1¼ to 2½+; large - 2½ to 3¼+.
(Feed twice a day)

Basic Homemade Meal for Liver Disease

Use this recipe and variations of it while toxins in the blood are high. This is the safest recipe with the highest nutritional value and easiest on the liver.

¼ **Cup non-fat cottage cheese**

¼ **Cup hard or medium tofu**
½ **Tablespoon extra virgin olive oil**

¼ **Cup cooked macaroni**

Cup raw or steamed mixed
¼ **vegetables (alfalfa sprouts, carrots, celery, artichoke heart)**
¼ **Cup water**

Substitutes:
Substitute ¼ cup of soy granules for tofu.
Substitute non-fat plain yogurt for the cottage cheese.
Substitute ½ cup cooked (boiled) liver for the cottage cheese and tofu.
Substitute ¼ cup of microwaved potatoes or yams (with the skin) for the macaroni.
Substitute 1 tablespoon of chopped raw almond slices for oil.

Vegetable preparation:
Wash and chop enough sprouts, celery and artichoke heart for 1 day (about ½ cup total) into bite-size pieces.
Steam or boil about ½ cup of peas and chopped carrots as directed. Combine all vegetables in container.

Enticers:
Add 4 tablespoons of chicken or beef broth.

1. Cook 1 cup of macaroni as directed on package. Allow to cool before serving.

2. Chop and prepare mixed vegetables.
3. Warm water in the microwave for 30 sec.
4. Combine cottage cheese, tofu, macaroni, vegetables, water and oil in food bowl.
5. Add digestive aid and medication as directed into meal and serve.
Store the unused vegetables and macaroni in separate containers and refrigerate.

Yield: *1 meal for medium size dog.*

Serving suggestions (in cups):
small — ¾ to 1¾; medium — 1¾ to 2½+; large - 2½ to 3¼+. (Feed 3-4 times a day)

Reheat:
Place serving of macaroni and vegetables in microwave-safe bowl and warm for 30 seconds or just long enough to reach room temperature. Then combine with the rest of the ingredients to prepare one meal.

Vegetable substitutes:
Feel free to substitute any of the vegetables with other vegetables on the list of healthy foods. Always use at least 3 different kinds for a total of 1 cup. Serve only ¼ cup in each meal.

Healthy Chicken, Vegetable, Pasta Stew
Use this recipe after blood levels return to normal.

1   Whole chicken or 5 lbs. of chicken pieces
1   Chopped yellow squash
1   Chopped zucchini
1   Chopped carrot
1   Cup chopped celery
2   Cups frozen green beans
1   Cup frozen baby green peas
1   Cup uncooked curly (Ritoni) pasta
1   Gallon of water
2   Tablespoons dried kelp (optional)

2   Teaspoons minced garlic (about 2 cloves)
2   Tablespoons dried basil or chopped fresh basil

Vegetable preparation:
Wash and chop fresh vegetables into bite-size pieces.
Vegetable substitutes:
Feel free to substitute any of the vegetables with other vegetables on the list of healthy foods. Always use at least 3 different kinds for a total of 4 cups.
Meat substitutes:
You can add ½ pound of chicken liver for added taurine and vitamins.
Meal variations:
Add ¼ cup of microwaved potatoes (with skin).
Reheat:
Put serving in microwave safe bowl and warm for 30 seconds or just long enough to reach room temperature.

1. In a large saucepan over medium-high heat, bring ½ gallon of water and chicken to a boil. Boil for 5-10 minutes while removing fat from the water.
2. Once the fat is cooked off the chicken, add 1 tablespoon of garlic, basil, and kelp.
3. Simmer chicken on low for at least 1 hour or until completely cooked. Remove chicken from bones and chop into bite-size pieces. Discard most of the skin and fat.
4. While chicken is cooking - In a large saucepan over medium-high heat, bring ½ gallon of water, pasta and vegetables to boil.
5. Add 1 tablespoon of garlic, basil and kelp to vegetables and pasta.
6. Simmer pasta and vegetables on low for 10 minutes. Remove from heat and keep covered until chicken is fully cooked.
7. Allow to cool before serving.
8. Mix one serving of vegetable pasta and chicken together with some broth.
9. Add digestive aid and medication before serving as directed.
Store the unused vegetables with pasta (together) and the chicken in broth separately in containers and refrigerate.

Yield: *About 8 cups of vegetables/pasta and 2 cups of chicken.*
Serving suggestions (in cups):
small – ½ to ¾; medium – 1 to 1½+; large 1½ to 2+.
(Feed 3-4 times a day.)
Ratio *of vegetable pasta to chicken: 2:1*
Example of 1 serving for a medium-size dog: ½ cup of vegetable pasta and ¼ cup of chicken (adjust as needed).

BULK, Healthy Chicken, Vegetable, Pasta Stew

Use this bulk recipe after you are sure it works for your dog and you want to save time preparing meals.

2	Large whole chickens or 10 lbs. of chicken pieces (like boneless, skinless thighs or breasts)	1. In a large stockpot over medium-high heat, bring 1 gallon of water and chicken to a boil. Boil for 5-10 minutes while removing fat from the water.
2	16-oz. bags of sliced yellow squash	2. Once the fat is cooked off the chicken, add 1½ tablespoons of garlic, basil, and kelp.
1	16-oz. bag of sliced carrot	3. Simmer chicken on low for at least 1 hour or until completely cooked.
2	16-oz. bags of frozen green beans	Remove chicken from bones and chop into bite-size pieces. Discard most of the skin and fat.
1	16-oz. bag of frozen baby green peas	4. In a large stock pot over medium-high heat, bring 1 gallon of water, pasta and vegetables to boil.
1	10-oz. bag of uncooked Rotini pasta	5. Add 1½ tablespoons of garlic, basil and kelp to vegetables and pasta.
2	Gallons of water	6. Simmer pasta and vegetables on low for 10 minutes. Remove from heat and keep covered until chicken is fully cooked.
3	Tablespoons garlic powder	7. Allow to cool before serving.
3	Tablespoons dried basil	8. Mix one serving of vegetables/pasta and chicken together with some broth.
3	Tablespoons dried kelp (optional)	9. Add digestive aid and medication before serving as directed.

Vegetable substitutes: Feel free to substitute any of the vegetables with other vegetables on the list of healthy foods. Always use at least 3 different kinds.

Store the unused vegetables with pasta (together) and chicken (in broth) separately in containers and freeze.

Meat substitutes: You can add 1 pound of chicken liver for added taurine and vitamins.

Yield: *About 22 cups of vegetables/pasta and 6 cups of chicken.*

Reheat: Put serving in microwave-safe bowl and warm for 30 seconds or just long enough to reach room temperature.

Serving suggestions (in cups): *small — ½ to ¾; medium — 1 to 1½+; large - 1½ to 2+. (Feed 3-4 times a day.)*

Ratio *of vegetable pasta to chicken: 2:1 Example of 1 serving for a medium size dog: ½ cup of vegetable pasta and ¼ cup of chicken (adjust as needed).*

43

Dr Dodd's Liver Cleansing Diet

This liver cleansing diet has been formulated by W. Jean Dodds, DVM. Dr. Dodds recommends a formula of 2 cups of cod fillet to 6 cups of veggies and potatoes, or 25% cod fillet to 75% veggies and potatoes.

1½ **Cups of new white potatoes**

1½ **Cups of sweet potatoes**

1½ **Cups of zucchini**

1½ **Cups of string beans, celery or summer squash**

2 **Cups of cod fillet**

1. Wash the potatoes well and cut them up crosswise into 2" pieces.

2. Simmer for 45 minutes to 1 hour and remove the skins.

3. Wash the zucchini and cut up with string beans, celery or squash and steam or cook until very tender.

4. Poach cod fillet in a frying pan with water until fish is white.

5. Combine and mix until well blended.

6. Mix one serving with digestive aid and medication as directed and serve.

Store the unused food in containers and refrigerate enough for 2 days. Freeze the rest.

Yield: *8 cups of food*

Serving suggestions (in cups):
small – ¾ to 1¾; medium – 1¾ to 2½+; large - 2½ to 3¼+.
(Feed 3-4 times a day)

Fast, Fresh Homemade Dog Food

Use this recipe when you suddenly discover that you are all out of your regular homemade dog food. This recipe should not be served on a regular basis. Use up to two or three times a week.

1   **Egg**
½   **Cup of cooked potatoes**
½   **Tablespoon extra virgin olive oil**

Substitutes:
You can substitute ½ cup of cooked macaroni or yams for the potatoes.

1. Lightly scramble egg in extra virgin olive oil.

2. Microwave 1 potato for 5 minutes.

3. Chop cooked potato into bite-size pieces.

4. Combine scrambled egg and ½ cup potatoes in food bowl. Allow to cool.

5. Add digestive aid and medication as directed into meal and serve.

Yield: *1 meal for medium-size dog.*

Serving suggestions (in cups): *small – ¾ to 1¾; medium – 1¾ to 2½+; large - 2½ to 3¼+.*
(Feed 2-3 times a day)

Chapter 5 – Supplements for Treating Liver Disease

"There is no doubt that God created these plants for our use, and gave certain individuals the talent for prescribing them, and promised us 'a land where …you will lack nothing.' (Deuteronomy 8:7)"
— Mary Ellen Hittinger

In addition to dietary therapy, supplementation is usually necessary. Check with your Vet to determine the individual needs of your dog.

Milk Thistle's Silymarin

Key role in curing Liver Disease

- Milk Thistle works to help the liver in 3 ways:
    1) It is a powerful antioxidant, which protects the body from free radicals. Free radicals can do damage to cells and eventually lead to cancer.
    2) It protects the liver from harmful toxins to prevent liver poisoning, helps treat liver diseases (of various kinds, including cirrhosis, chronic hepatitis, fatty infiltration of the liver and inflammation of the bile duct) and improves liver function.
    3) It helps the liver regenerate itself by stimulating the growth of liver cells to replace the cells that are damaged.
- Even extreme cases of hepatitis and liver degeneration have shown improvement when treated with Milk Thistle.
- Milk Thistle is the most researched and best understood of all medicinal herbs.
- Studies have confirmed Milk Thistle's ability to protect and rejuvenate the liver.
- Milk Thistle is even more potent when taken with other herbs, such as dandelion, artichoke and licorice. (This complex is known as Milk Thistle X.) This combination enhances liver protection and bile excretion.

- Silymarin cannot cure cirrhosis, which is a very destructive form of liver disease, but it can support the part of the liver that is still healthy and working.
- Milk Thistle has been found to prevent or reduce medication-induced liver damage.
- Milk Thistle is very safe to take and does not have any negative effects, even when taken in high doses over a long period of time.
- Silymarin is many times more potent in antioxidant activity than Vitamin E and Vitamin C.
- You can find Milk Thistle (Silymarin) at your local health food store. Make sure Silymarin, or Silybum Marianum, is listed in the ingredients in a standardized formula with at least 80% Silymarin. There are several producers and four basic formulas to choose from:
  1) Milk Thistle in capsule formula (dosage 150 mg per capsule).
  2) Milk Thistle X (Milk Thistle, Dandelion, Artichoke, and Licorice) capsule formula (dosage 150 mg per capsule).
  3) Liver Tonic in a liquid herbal extract formula, which contains a mixture of Milk Thistle, Dandelion Root and other beneficial herbs.
  4) Super Milk Thistle has a new form of Silymarin that is bound to phosphatidylcholine. The bound version of Silymarin is more effective than the unbound version. This new formula also has Dandelion, like Milk Thistle X.

Healing Herbs and Supplements

This table of herbs and supplements includes essential, important and helpful supplements that can be given with the Healthy Homemade Dog Food for the treatment of liver disease and cirrhosis.

Check with your Vet before starting any of these supplements to make sure they are right for your dog. The dosages given are guidelines. Ask your Vet about the right dosage for your dog.

Supplement	Benefits and Comments	Suggested Dosage	Safety Issues
Vital			
Milk Thistle (Silymarin)	Has been shown to repair and rejuvenate the liver.	100mg per 25lb, 2-3x/day	None
Vitamin E (Use d-alpha-tocopherol form)	Protects from metabolism of cell membranes. Powerful antioxidant, aids circulation.	200 IU per day	High doses have a "blood-thinning" effect.
Vitamin B complex	Needed for digestion and nutrient absorption, brain function, appetite, and formation of red blood cells.	50mg 2x/day	None
Vitamin B12	Prevents anemia, protects nerves.	22mkg of food/day	None
Omega-3 Fatty Acids (fish oil, flax seed oil)	Anti-oxidant, anti-inflammatory Helps liver, joint, brain function, and protects the circulatory system.	Unknown see your Vet.	High doses have a "blood-thinning" effect.
Valuable			
L-Carnitine	Used to turn fat into energy. May be helpful for pets with cognitive disorder (senility). Liver disease may inhibit carnitine production. Helps prevent build-up of fat in liver. Antioxidant, protects against cancer in liver.	500 mg 2x/day on empty stomach	Rare side effects – diarrhea, intestinal gas.
Taurine	The most essential antioxidant. Protects from damage of free radicals.	500mg 2-3x/day	None.
Alpha-Lipoic acid	Powerful antioxidant. Helps balance levels of sugar in the blood.	100 mg 1x/day	None.
Dandelion root	Useful for stimulating liver circulation, bile production, as a diuretic, to improve digestion, eliminate waste, and as an anti-inflammatory.	Unknown. see your Vet.	Not for pets on hypoglycemic therapy, with gallbladder disease or bile duct obstruction.

Supplement	Benefits and Comments	Suggested Dosage	Safety Issues
Useful			
Vitamin C	Liver Disease may decrease the amount of Vitamin C in the system.	200 mg 1x/day	Long-term use could cause kidney stones. High doses may cause diarrhea.
L-Arginine	Helps detoxify ammonia, produced in the digestion of protein. It can build up when the liver isn't properly functioning.	500mg 1x/day on empty stomach	None.
Choline (or lecithin)	Helps liver and gallbladder functioning and regulation. A powerful fat emulsifier. Especially recommended for pets with fatty liver disease.	1,200 ppm with meal	Rare side effects – anemia.
Garlic (allium)	Detoxifies liver, bloodstream.	1 raw clove per day or 10 mg of allium daily with meal.	Too much is toxic. Not for pets with anemia or if surgery is scheduled. Stop use within a minimum of 1 week before and after surgery. May cause excessive intestinal gas.
Free-form amino acid complex	A good protein source that is gentle on the liver.	Unknown see your Vet.	Unknown.

Supplement	Benefits and Comments	Suggested Dosage	Safety Issues
Turmeric	A powerful antioxidant, has protective effects on the liver, like Silymarin, and beneficial effects on the gastrointestinal tract including decreased gas formation and spasm.	1 tsp/day	Do not use in pets with bile duct obstruction, gallbladder stones or gastrointestinal upset.
Grape seed extract	Antioxidant. Helps liver to cleanse the body of toxic substances.	Unknown see your Vet.	Unknown.
Selenium	Good detoxifier and natural antioxidant that works with Vitamin E.	0.11 mg/ kg of food	Safe at recommended doses.
Zinc	Needed for immune system and healing functions.	100mg 2x/ day for 3-6 months then 50mg 2x/day on empty stomach	Long-term side effects – copper deficiency, decreased immunity, heart problems, anemia. Can interfere in soy, manganese, penicillamine and tetracycline absorption.
Bonemeal (tablets or human grade powder)	To promote healing of tissue and provide calcium and phosphorus.	¾ - 1 tsp per day or 3-4 tablets per day	Avoid if your dog has skeletal problems, cancer, parathyroid gland problems, kidney or bladder stones or if taking antibiotics, and other pain medications. Check with your vet if you're not sure.

Health Fact
Milk Thistle's Silymarin not only protects the liver from harmful toxins, it actually helps the liver regenerate itself by stimulating the growth of liver cells to replace the parts of the liver that are damaged. Super Milk Thistle, with a bound version of Silymarin, is even more effective than the unbound version.

Multi-Vitamin, Dietary Supplement & Digestive Enzymes

Multi-Vitamin

To ensure proper balance of all the vitamins and minerals, add a high quality, complete multi-vitamin and mineral supplement. You can use a natural, raw human vitamin-mineral supplement, although a better natural product suited for your dog is Canine Plus by Vetri-Science.

Follow your Vets' advice when choosing a vitamin-mineral supplement. Just like not all human vitamins are of the same quality, not all dog vitamins are the same. You want the best- quality product with all the vitamins, antioxidants and minerals you can get to help restore your dog's health. You aren't giving your dog a vitamin to maintain health; you're giving it to him to restore his health. Don't skip this important part. This is NOT Optional! **Without a good multi-vitamin your Healthy Homemade Dog Food can be unbalanced and cause more health problems.**

Dietary Supplement

The Missing Link® is a dietary supplement designed to deliver the perfect ratio of essential omega oils in combination with a broad spectrum of natural fiber, flaxseed lignans, phytonutrients, and more. The whole foods and food concentrates are not processed or altered. They provide added natural nutritional benefits when coupled with any animal food available (dry food, raw diet, home prepared, etc).

Flaxseed is the primary ingredient along with bone meal, fish meal, liver, oyster, whey protein and more. This dietary supplement has been used by veterinarians and pet owners for years. The Missing Link® can be used instead of the homemade Healthy Powder and in addition to any other supplement you are giving your dog.

Digestive Enzymes

Digestive enzymes are required for a variety of functions. Enzymes aid in food digestion, absorption and maximize the utilization of nutrients found in natural raw diets. Prozyme © and Shake-N-Zyme © are two recommended plant enzyme supplements that have proven beneficial for dogs. One of these products or a similar product is usually available from your Vet.

Avoid These

It is just as important to know what NOT to give your dog, as it is to know what to give your dog. You want to avoid all toxic substances. Here are a few key items you want to avoid exposing your dog to.

Foods to Avoid
- Fried or grilled meat and bones
- Sugar
- Chocolate
- Onion
- Citrus fruit
- Nightshade family: Bella Donna, egg-plant, tomatoes, both red and green bell peppers (so, no pizza)
- Dog treats and bones

Household Items to Avoid
- Plastic food bowl (stainless steel bowls are best)
- Pesticides
- Smoking
- Aromatherapy Oils

Medications to Avoid
- NSAID's like Ibuprofen, Acetaminophen, Rimadyl, or Aspirin
- Flea & Tick Medications (unless absolutely necessary)
- Heartworm Preventative (unless absolutely necessary)
- Vaccinations (that aren't required)

- Steroids, Antibiotics and other medications that have liver failure side-effects (if prescribed by your Vet ask for safer alternatives and monitor blood levels closely)

Pet Items to Avoid

- Flea & Tick Dips and Shampoos
- Flea Collars

Chapter 6 – Caring for Your Sick Dog

"Dogs laugh, but they laugh with their tails." – Max Eastman

Taking care of a sick dog with liver disease is not for the meek or the very busy. You may need to adjust your schedule and life-style to make time to cook, feed, take trips outside, give love and affection and go to the Vet. But, I assume you love your dog very much, or you wouldn't be reading this book. Keep a positive attitude and know that you are doing everything you can to save your dog's life.

Part of caring for your sick dog includes:
- Regular trips to the Vet
- Watching for symptoms of progressing liver disease
- Potty patrol
- Quick check-ups
- Giving your dog pills
- Bathing
- Controlling your emotions, and more…

This chapter will give you guidance on how to best care for your sick dog.

Good Veterinary Care

It's very important to have a good Vet who believes in using homemade diets, alternative medicine, supplements, food remedies and even holistic care. Decide what you want from your Vet and go looking for it. (see More Resources for AHVMA website of Holistic Vets in your area)

Now that you know what you want, make a list of questions to ask your potential Vet. Interview them before you go see them. Make sure they answer your questions and are willing to work closely with you in the care and treatment of your dog with liver disease.

You will be seeing your Vet on a regular basis, so you want to make sure that you will get the type of treatment you need and have all your questions answered to your satisfaction.

Communication from Your Dog

One of the hardest parts about caring for a sick dog is not knowing what's wrong. Since they can't tell you what hurts or what's wrong, you'll need to learn how your dog communicates symptoms.

Everything your dog does is communicating something to you. In the following sections, you'll learn what some of those things mean and what you should be looking out for.

These are some of the common signs and symptoms that you will be looking out for:
- Diarrhea – straining / stool color / blood / mucus.
- Vomiting – color / mucoid / foamy / time-lapse after eating / time of day or night.
- Urination Accidents (or frequent urination)
- House Soiling Accidents
- Begging, Demanding Attention or Acting Very Needy
- Changes in Behaviors – wandering off, seizures, aimless pacing or circling, head pressing.
- Changes in Temperament / Alertness – decreased activity, awareness of surroundings.
- Changes in Eating - eating grass, eating charcoal, seems hungry all the time (ravenous appetite), no appetite, eating own stool or other unusual objects.
- Changes in Sleeping Habits – lays down in different spot, restless and can't sleep, or sleeps constantly.
- Signs of Progressing Liver Disease – depression, swollen belly, jaundice (yellow eyes and skin), chronic weight loss.

Potty Patrol

First of all, you need to know that you're going to be on potty patrol from now on. That's right. You will be looking at your dog's stool. The stool is a major indicator of how your dog is doing. It will tell you how your dog's digestion is going, how much the liver is processing, or not processing and a whole lot more. Get in the habit of watching your dog potty. Notice the amount, color, consistency, odor (if unusual) and frequency of your dog's stool. Watch for straining. If your dog has diarrhea (loose stools) for more than 2 or 3 days, or has diarrhea and vomiting, you will need to take action and see your Vet due to possible dehydration.

A normal stool is well-formed, or solid, with no mucus, blood or undigested food. Diarrhea can take on many forms and have many causes. The more specific you can be about the characteristics of your dog's diarrhea the better your Vet will be able to diagnose and treat the problem. Diarrhea is common when making drastic changes in your dog's diet. If you have not changed your dog's diet, something else could be wrong. Diarrhea is also a common side-effect of many drugs and medications, particularly the NSAID's (Non-Steroidal Anti-Inflammatory Drugs).

In diagnosing the cause of diarrhea, the Vet will need to decide whether the diarrhea originates in the small bowel or the large bowel. The characteristics of the diarrhea, as well as the condition of your dog, will help your Vet make this determination.

The following chart gives you an idea of what to look for and what your Vet may determine.

What diarrhea tells you about your dog

Characteristics of Diarrhea

Indicator	Problem	Part of Digestive System
Appearance		
Yellow, greenish, watery	Rapid transit through bowel	Small bowel
Black, dark blood	Bleeding of Upper GI tract	Stomach, small bowel
Red blood, clots	Bleeding of Lower GI tract	Colon, anus
Pasty, light	Bile Insufficiency	Liver, pancreas

Indicator	Problem	Part of Digestive System
Bulky, gray, containing un-digested food, like rice or carrots.	Insufficient digestion/ absorption	Small bowel, liver, pancreas
Loose, foamy	Intestinal bacteria infection	Small bowel
Oily	Poor food absorption	Small bowel, pancreas
Shiny or jellylike	Contains mucus	Colon
Odor		
Smelling like food or sour milk	Rapid transit through bowel and insufficient digestion/ absorption (likely due to overfeeding)	Small bowel, pancreas
Foul smelling	Insufficient digestion, sug-gests fermentation of stool	Small bowel, pancreas
Amount		
3-4 small stools within a short time, with straining	Inflammation of the Colon (Colitis)	Colon
3-4 bulky stools within 24 hours	Insufficient digestion/ absorption	Small bowel, pancreas
Changes in the Dog		
Weight loss	Insufficient digestion/ absorption	Small bowel, pancreas
Normal weight and appetite	Large bowel condition	Colon
Vomiting	Enteritis, Gastritis, Pancreatitis	Small bowel, stomach, colon (in rare cases)

(Adapted from Dog Owner's Home Veterinary Handbook)

Vomiting

Dogs are good at vomiting. Vomiting is very common and has many causes. However, sporadic vomiting that occurs off and on over a period of days or weeks, with no relationship to meals, may indicate that a chronic condition, such as liver disease, is present. Persistent vomiting or retches of a frothy, yellow or clear fluid could indicate a stomach problem, such as acute gastritis, which is a common liver disease-related illness.

When vomiting occurs, take note of the following to report to your Vet.

- Is the vomiting repeated? If so, does your dog vomit or retch repeatedly, bringing up a frothy, yellow or clear fluid? Or, does your dog vomit off and on over a period of days or weeks with no relationship to meals?
- Is there a relationship to meals? How soon after eating does it occur? Is it projectile (flying from mouth)?
- Inspect the vomitus for blood, food material – digested or undigested, fecal material, foreign objects and worms.

Urination Accidents

When a change in the frequency of urination occurs, these are clues to health problems. Increased thirst, or frequent drinking, and urination are signs of possible kidney failure or other metabolic disease. Too much protein in your dog's diet can cause your dog's kidneys to work overtime and begin to fail. Do not ignore this common symptom. Take your dog to see your Vet to determine the specific cause and treatment.

Soiling Accidents

There are several causes of house soiling. If the soiling is diarrhea, it could be a sign of an acute case of gastroenteritis, or other problem, and warrants a trip to the Vet. Soiling could also be due to failing memory or a cognitive problem. Do not punish your dog if this occurs. Most likely, the dog could not help himself. Scolding and punishment only produces fear and anxiety, which makes the problem worse.

Begging or Demanding Attention or Acting Very Needy

A behavioral change like begging for attention or comfort and acting very needy should not be ignored. This behavior suggests discomfort or pain, possibly associated with eating. When a behavioral change like this occurs, take note of the following:

- When does the need for attention or comfort happen? Is there a relationship to meals, say 1 or 2 hours after eating?
- Does your dog's stomach growl or get upset?
- Is your dog passing gas or constipated?
- Is your dog vomiting?
- Does your dog have diarrhea?

Changes in Behavior
Wandering Off

If your dog starts to behave differently, like wandering off or forgetting where you are, this is a sign of cognitive problems. Some supplements help support cognitive functions and can slow down mental deterioration. (See Supplements with cognitive support.)

Changes in Eating Habits
Eating Grass or Other Unusual Objects, Ravenous Appetite, Loss of Appetite

When your dog eats grass or charcoal, that could be an indication of an upset stomach. Upset stomach can occur because of something as simple as your dog raiding the garbage can, or because of bad meat in the last meal. If this persists over several days, it could be a sign of something more serious and you should see your Vet.

If your dog starts eating stools, there could be a medical problem or nutritional deficiency. If your dog has a ravenous appetite, he could be eating stools in an attempt to acquire additional calories. Add small amounts of protein and carbohydrates, or break the meal up into small portions and increase the number of feedings. If this does not stop the behavior, ask your Vet about it. There could be a problem with food processing or absorption.

If your dog has an upset stomach, he may stop eating. This is a normal response. It allows the digestive system to get back to normal. Give him broth and water to help keep him hydrated while his system gets reset.

If your dog's appetite does not improve within 24 hours, this is cause for alarm. Take him in to the Vet to make sure he doesn't get dehydrated and to diagnose the problem.

Changes in Sleeping Habits

Lays down in different spot, Restlessness, Sleeplessness, Increased or Decreased Sleeping

Where your dog lays down and sleeps can actually tell you a lot about what kind of mood he's in. Think about where your dog usually lies down during different times of the day. Does he have favorite spots? Notice if these spots of the house are colder or warmer than other spots or areas. Does he lie down in a place near you or away from you?

If your dog starts lying down in a different place, and that place is away from you, this could mean he's not feeling good. The contrary is also true. As long as he's lying down in the same spots as usual, and those spots are near you, this is a good sign that he's feeling good.

A change is sleeping patterns can also tell you when your dog doesn't feel good. If he's restless at night, or waking you up to let him out, it could be a sign of discomfort. This usually goes along with other changes like diarrhea and vomiting. Likewise, a good night's sleep can be a good sign that he's feeling good. However, sleeping all the time or more than usual could also be a sign of problems.

Signs of Progressing Liver Disease

Depression, Swollen Belly, Jaundice (yellow eyes and skin), Chronic Weight Loss

It is very important to stay on the lookout for signs that the liver disease is progressing. If the original symptoms do not go away, and these signs appear, the Liver is not responding or regenerating with the treatment.

Let's look at each of the signs individually.

Depression

If your dog does not want to play or refuses to go for walks, or lies down in a different spot and stays there for most of the time, these are signs of depression or lethargy. This should be watched carefully to see if it progresses.

Swollen Belly (Ascites)

If your dog has a swollen belly that looks like it's full of fluid, this is known as ascites. This could be a liver or circulation (heart) problem.

Jaundice (yellow eyes, gums, and skin)

If the whites of your dogs eyes begin to yellow this could be because the liver is not processing properly. The gums and skin may also appear yellow.

Chronic Weight Loss

If your dog has little or no appetite, or a good or ravenous appetite and is still losing weight, this is a sign that the liver is failing to process all the nutritional building blocks and the body is failing to maintain itself. This condition is known as *wasting*.

Special Needs of Dogs with Liver Disease

When dogs are seriously ill, they need to go off by themselves to rest and allow nature to heal the condition. They often stop eating and lie down in a cozy place that is quiet and out of the way. This gives your dog a sense of security. Allow your dog to be off by himself, but offer reassurance and comfort that you love him and are there for him. Don't try to force your dog to eat right away or to come out and play. Be patient, but watchful.

Fasting

Fasting is good for your dog. It gives the digestive system a break, and the liver a chance to eliminate toxins and expel wastes that build up within. This cleansing process is especially important for dogs with liver disease. Fasting for one day a week is recommended as a regular part of treating liver disease while your dog is in the first stages of recovery (while blood tests show liver disease is present). Fasting should not be done if your dog is hypoglycemic. Consult with your Vet before beginning a fasting regimen.

- Use a 24-hour broth fast to give your dog something to drink that doesn't need to be digested and processed.
- Start the fast in the morning with a cup of water and 2-4 tablespoons of beef or chicken broth (low-sodium). Continue giving broth in place of each meal until the next morning.
- Try to prepare your own meals quickly or in advance to avoid smelling up the house with food your dog can't eat.
- Don't leave your dog alone all day when you have him on a fast.
- Give extra love and attention during normal feeding times to help him feel cared for and not punished.
- After the fast, if your dog has trouble having bowel movements you can help get things going by increasing the amount of insoluble fiber (like sweet potatoes, prunes, fruit or raw celery) in the diet. Note that it will take several hours for your dog to resume his regular potty schedule.

How to Give Your Dog a Quick Check-up

It's important to keep a close eye on your dog's state to make sure the liver disease is not progressing. Keep a look out for all of the common symptoms of liver disease as well as pigmentation changes (turning yellow), bruising, excessive redness, uncontrolled bleeding and signs of pain.

By examining your dog regularly, you can monitor his overall health and track the progress of treatment. Perform this quick check-up weekly at first and then monthly after your dog has stabilized. Be sure to resolve any concerns with your Vet.

Adapted from Dr. Pitcairn's Complete Guide to Natural Health for Dogs & Cats.

1) Examine the eyes. Check for matter in the corners. Gently pull down the lower eyelids so you can see the whites of the eye. Do the whites look yellow, bruised, have popped blood vessels or look red? If yes, your dog may have jaundice – contact your Vet for treatment.

2) Look in the ear holes. Do you see wax? Do the insides look oily? Sniff to check for an offensive odor. Does the skin pigmentation look yellow or have excessive redness? Does your dog react in pain when touching the ear? If yes, contact your Vet.

3) Check the gums and teeth. Gently raise the upper lip and push back the corners of the lips at the same time. You don't need to open the mouth. Do the gums have a red line along the roots of the teeth? Do the gums look yellow, white, bruised or bleeding? Are the teeth gleaming white or coated with brown deposits? Smell the breath. Does it smell okay, or are you overcome by it? Is there saliva in the mouth, or is your dog drooling? If yes, contact your Vet.

4) Run your hand along the hair coat back and forth – with and against the grain. Does the coat feel greasy? Do you see dandruff or little black specks? Black specks are the excreta of fleas. Smell your hand. Does it smell like "dog odor", is it rancid, rank or fishy? Is your dog losing hair or excessively shedding? If so, it's a sign of poor health due to liver disease or another medical condition. Starting a new diet may also trigger a cleansing process that could cause an odor during detoxification.

5) Pull up on the skin and let go. Does the skin stay sticking up? If so, your dog is dehydrated. See your Vet for treatment. Do you notice any pigmentation or color change? Is the skin yellow or bruised? Are there any sores or spots that may have been bleeding? These are all signs of liver disease. If you notice any changes, contact your Vet.

6) Last, feel the backbone in the middle of the back. Do you feel defined bones there? Is there a prominent ridge sticking up in the middle? If so, your dog is much too thin, and this could be a sign of wasting.

Don't forget about Potty Patrol. Also, watch how many times and how long your dog urinates. To measure how much your dog urinates, just count (one one-hundred, two one-hundred...) while he urinates. Look at the color of the urine. Make sure it's not orange or red. Also, watch for straining to urinate or potty.

Creative Ways to Give Your Dog a Pill

You are going to be giving your dog at least one pill a day, possibly a handful several times a day. Instead of the traditional method of opening your dog's mouth and inserting the pill down the throat and inducing swallowing, here are a few creative ways to make this easy for you and your dog.

Since most dogs do not chew their food, it's easy to hide pills in some favorite foods that your dog will eat without question.

- Start by giving your dog the pill-hiding food by itself, as a treat, to make sure your dog likes it.
- Then give your dog a pill that is hidden in the food along with some more of the pill-hiding food, again like you would give him a treat.
- After a few days of hiding the pill you can try just putting the pill in your hand, or a small dish, and covering over it with a little pill-hiding food to see if he will eat them along with the food.
- Once your dog is used to this new treat, you can put several pills in your hand at once and cover them with the pill-hiding food. Your dog will eat the handful of pills and food like a treasured treat and never know the difference.

Some good pill-hiding healing foods are:
- Prunes
- Raspberries
- Banana
- Cheese

Bathing and Grooming

Continue to give your dog a regular bath and trim the nails to keep your dog clean and healthy. Use an oatmeal based shampoo and conditioner, or whatever your Vet indicates for hair and skin health. If you use a dog Groomer, ask them to withhold any perfumes, and DO NOT dip your dog for fleas.

Non-Toxic Flea & Tick Control

Do not use any flea & tick control dips, sprays, powders, collars or shampoos until your dog's health has been built up through the homemade liver diet and supplements. Then, use only non-toxic, or the least toxic, and most natural flea & tick control program.

Start your flea and tick control program with these non-toxic steps adapted from *Dr. Pitcairn's Complete guide to Natural Health for Dogs & Cats.*

- Steam clean your carpets at the first site of fleas and ticks to kill flea eggs before they hatch.
- Vacuum and clean the floors and furniture where your dog sleeps at least once a week to pickup flea eggs, larvae and pupae. Immediately dispose of vacuum bag or its contents to prevent escape. Or, clean the outdoor doghouse to get rid of fleas and their eggs.
- Launder your dog's bedding at least once a week in hot, soapy water and dry on maximum heat.
- Bathe your dog in a natural non-toxic flea & tick control shampoo.
- Brush your dog with a flea comb to trap and kill fleas already on your dog.
- Mow and water your lawn regularly to drown developing fleas and ticks.
- Do not use pesticides that kill all insects in your yard, especially ants. Ants eat flea eggs and larvae. Beneficial nematodes are an alternative to pesticides and are available at most nurseries.
- Add garlic to your dog's diet.

Heart Worm Preventative

Do not use Heart Worm preventative until your dog's health has been built up and blood levels are back to normal. If you do use a Heart Worm preventative, watch for signs of a relapse.

Vaccinations

Stop all vaccinations until your dog is stabilized. Then discuss with your Vet to determine what is absolutely necessary. Ask your Vet about nosodes, the vaccine alternative. If you do vaccinate your dog, give extra doses of Milk Thistle before and after the vaccination, followed by a checkup one week later to look for any signs of a reaction or decline in health.

Emotional Health

It's important to pay special attention to emotional issues in your home to foster a positive emotional climate and help your dog heal. Your dog's health is affected by feelings of tension, anxiety, depression, anger and other emotional upsets in the home. Your attitude and expectations about liver disease will have a pronounced effect on the outcome. To promote emotional health and healing:

- Begin to notice how your dog reacts to your emotions and emotions in your home.
- Reassure and give extra positive attention and love, when you and your dog are in a good mood, to support emotional health and healing.
- Have faith in the power of healing. Pray for guidance in selecting your dog's healthcare practitioner, wisdom to take good care of your dog and for your dog's healing.
- Treat your dog like an older puppy, not a sick dog.
- Don't scold or punish your dog for accidents, house soiling, or begging for attention. Give extra love and attention using a positive tone of voice.
- Don't worry about your dog's health. Be grateful and thankful for everyday you have with him.
- Eliminate as much stress as you can from your life. From this point forward be as relaxed, confident and calm as possible.

When upset, avoid interaction with your dog and family members. Take a break when you need it to gain a fresh perspective.

- Use alternative treatments to reduce your stress. Some good ones to try are Bach Flower Remedies, Aromatherapy and Music therapy.

(Dr. Pitcairn's Complete Guide to Natural Health for Dogs & Cats)

Author Aleithia Artemis, an Animal Behavior/Emotions Specialist and long-time studier of health-related influences, has this advice:

"Positive emotional attention must be given exclusively when both you and your dog are in a *good mood* (or at least a neutral one) *to begin with.* *Nonchalance* (or at least its appearance) should be given when you or your dog are stressed. Obvious exception: dire emergency. That IS the proper time to panic, and rush to one's chosen health care practitioner. There's a time for everything under the sun, and yes, sometimes panicking is the responsible thing to do.

The idea to keep in mind: When you are feeling panic-stricken over the looming prospect of losing your best friend and unconditional lover; but the situation truly is not an emergency – separate yourself from your dog and pretend nonchalance, while you administer your own needed emotional self-care. When you return to sanity, go back and enjoy your dog. They are, after all, STILL ALIVE WITH YOU HERE AND NOW. Concentrate on and savor the goodness of that truth."

Chapter 7 – Liver Related Illnesses and Treatment

"Homeopathy cures a greater percentage of cases than any other method of treatment. Homeopathy is the latest [most] refined method of treating patients economically and non-violently." – Mahatma Gandhi

Liver Disease can create other problems that you must treat as they arise. One common illness is Gastritis, or stomach problems.

Gastritis or Stomach Problems

The common signs of stomach problems are poor digestion (undigested food in the stool, large more frequent stools), vomiting and diarrhea, gas, growling stomach, eating grass or charcoal, depression, hiding (either immediately after eating or an hour or so later), loss of appetite or acting very needy. The common causes of stomach problems are spoiled food, excessive grains, fermented grains, food allergies, eating raw bones and intestinal parasites.

The two most common forms of stomach problems are Acute Gastritis (sudden upset) and Chronic Gastritis (low-grade, persistent upset). Usually the underlying cause will need to be determined.

Dr. Pitcairn's Complete Guide to Natural Health for Dogs & Cats gives several homeopathic treatments for both acute and chronic gastritis. The right treatment to use is determined by identifying the specific symptoms and using the treatment that works best for each symptom. The symptoms can be from multiple or varying causes, which may need to be determined specifically to treat effectively.

A good first step is to withhold food for 12-24 hours to allow rest and healing. A clear broth fast is a good way to do this.

For the dog that wants attention and comfort (acts needy), especially if he is not interested in drinking, you should try an Antacid or Kaopectate®. Give your dog one chewable tablet. It is safe to use with liver disease, and it is very effective for relieving upset stomach, indigestion and diarrhea associated with Acute or Chronic Gastritis.

Another treatment is a Homeopathic Remedy – *Pulsatilla 12C (wind-flower)*. Dogs that require this remedy often become ill by eating food that is rich or fatty. Adjust the diet to reduce the amount of fat. Homeopathic remedies are very different from conventional medicine. They do not work as effectively if they are given with food. They are administered crushed. Grind the pellet and place in a bowl. (You may need to buy a pill crusher.) Then let your dog lick the crushed pellet out of the bowl. The powder will be absorbed in the mouth, bypassing the digestive system.

For Acute Gastritis give one pellet every 4 hours until the symptoms are gone. Do not feed your dog for fifteen minutes before and after treatment. If your dog shows signs of improvement, continue giving the treatment for five days. Discontinue as soon as the symptoms are completely gone. If you do not see a response within 24 hours, you should take your dog to the Vet.

For Chronic Gastritis that shows up in the dog that has a good appetite but gets upset with changes in the diet, or is prone to gas and constipation, give digestive enzymes with food and look for food sensitivities. Remove any food items from the diet that are on the list of common food allergies.

You could also try an Herbal Remedy – *Garlic (Allium sativum)*. For strictly stomach problems, give ½ teaspoon to 1 tablespoon of garlic extract 3 times a day until the problem is relieved. Make garlic extract by soaking 4 to 6 chopped cloves in ½ cup of cold water for 8 hours and then strain. For intestinal problems give 1 garlic softgel capsule a day with a meal until symptoms are gone. If problems recur, you may want to add this to your daily regimen.

You can also use *Pulsatilla* for chronic gastritis. The main difference with acute and chronic gastritis is that the chronic form of illness has less intense symptoms as the acute stage. For example, your dog may be "clingy", wanting attention and drinking less water, but not vomiting or showing signs of diarrhea. Chronic symptoms do not stand out as strongly as when they are seen in the acute form.

Although it is common for dogs to have an upset stomach, make sure there is not some other underlying cause. If chronic symptoms do not go away, it may be time to see your Vet.

Allergies/Sensitivities

Allergies are a common condition that you may run across. It's important for you to know the common symptoms of allergies, so that you can search for the cause and not just treat the symptom. Once you start using the recipes in this book and creating your own diet, you will want to stay on the look out for these symptoms, so you can identify food sensitivity as soon as it emerges. Then, of course, once you identify the food item that is causing the adverse reaction you will want to remove that item from all further recipes.

Symptoms of an Allergic Reaction

- Scratching – caused by itchy skin or eruptions, especially on the lower back near the base of the tail, or anywhere and everywhere on the body.
- Inflamed ears.
- Excessive licking of the front legs and top of the paw.
- Digestive upsets (gurgling, gas and a tendency toward diarrhea).
- Inflammation of the toes.
- Irritated rear end (anus, anal sacs and genitals) with licking and dragging of the rear on the floor.
- Itchy eyes with gook in the corners.

"Research suggests that about a third of all allergies are caused by substances in foods. You can easily identify the immediate trigger by using a [hypoallergenic] diet for a while. If the symptoms subside but return when you go back to the original diet, you can assume that your dog is allergic to one or more of the ingredients in the daily diet." (*Dr. Pitcairn's Complete Guide to Natural Health for Dogs & Cats*

71

Common Food Allergens

- Beef
- Wheat
- Rice
- Milk
- Cheese
- Eggs
- Nuts
- Fruits
- Tomatoes
- Carrots
- Yeast
- Various spices, additives, and dyes
- Flavorings in chewable vitamins
- Many others…

How to Determine Cause of Allergic Reaction

Determining exactly what is causing the allergic reaction can be difficult. Start with a basic diet with common food allergens omitted. Give the basic diet for an extended period of time (3-4 months). If the problem clears up or improves, slowly reintroduce the omitted foods, one at a time, to find out which one or ones are causing the problem. If the problem does not clear up with a basic diet, the cause may not be a food allergy. This is where things can get difficult or impossible. You may need to work with a trained professional to determine the exact cause of the allergy. Blood tests can also be run to determine the most likely foods your dog is sensitive to.

How to Control Allergies

To help control allergies, give high doses of Vitamin C, B-Complex, and Omega-3 Fatty Acids. They act as natural antihistamines. There are also some good Homeopathic Remedies for allergies. Consult with your Vet and check your local Health Food store to find one that works for your dog's specific allergies.

Chapter 8 – Gratitude and Faith

"Little miracles come into our lives, not on huge bolts of lightning, but on gentle beams of light, love and hope." – Dan Zadra

When I think back over the past year since Norman was first diagnosed, I am amazed at how far we two have come. I am filled with gratitude for every day I've had with Norman. When I look to the future, I have faith that this book will help many other dog lovers care for their beloved best friends. I know that Norman will not live forever. I have nearly faced his inevitable death twice now. Each time I let go a little more, learn a little more and feel even more grateful for each moment of each day that I still have him.

I'm not fighting with death anymore. I've faced my fears, acknowledged my feelings and learned tremendously from the deep emotions that come from the loss of a furry family member. Instead of fighting, I'm going with the flow of the river of life. Death is just a part of life. It comes to all of us. When it does come, I know I will be sad, disappointed, angry and even depressed. I will miss Norman terribly. He has been my companion and best friend for over 12 years. But, I'll be comforted in knowing that I didn't give up hope, and I did my best to care for him.

This Book is For You

This book took longer than I expected to finish. Doing the research to help Norman and writing it all down were two very different things. But, I have learned even more by taking the time to synthesize it. The hardest part of finishing this book was not knowing if I had done enough. I doubted my recipes and treatment. I didn't want to tell anyone to do something if I wasn't 100% sure it was right. Every time Norman got sick I would blame myself, and tell myself I was doing something wrong. For as long as he was sick, I couldn't finish the book. Then, when he had his last crisis, I didn't think he was going to make it. And that cast a big shadow of doubt on ever finishing it. But, he recovered and here I am, writing the last chapter. I was compelled to finish it today. I feel like I owe it to Norman. I'm also convinced that someone else is out there who desperately needs the information I have in this book, because their dog has just been diagnosed with liver disease. It may not be perfect, and it's definitely not everything there is to know about how to care for a dog with liver disease. But, it's a whole lot more than what was out there when I started looking over a year ago.

This book is written for you and the dog that you love. I hope you find it useful, informational and inspirational. I want it to give you hope for your dog's healing.

I encourage you to do your own research and develop your own homemade dog food that's just right for your dog. Remember, you know your dog better than anyone else does. Listen to your heart and follow common sense. Work with a Vet who supports alternative treatments. Get the resources you need to feel like you're doing your best. Everything you learn about how to care for your dog will improve your own well-being and your dog's quality of life.

Afterword

Update on Norman

The treatment described in this book healed Norman's drug induced liver disease in only three months. The diet, supplements and care supported his liver and organs.

I'm happy to say that, after 2 years from his initial diagnosis and prognosis of less than a month, Norman never had any liver disease symptoms again.

But, in addition to liver disease, Norman had severe arthritis. With the liver damage, Norman could not take any conventional pain medications. I continued my research on how to treat arthritis. I found several homeopathic alternatives and supplements that helped with pain. But throughout the year his arthritis just kept getting worse. I kept increasing his dosages for pain, but it would only help for a few days or weeks. Then I could see he was in pain again.

When the pain was bad, he could barely walk around, so I was carrying him everywhere. He could barely stand up long enough to eat. When it got so bad that he couldn't stand up on his own and needed help going outside to potty, I knew it was time to do something.

I considered getting him a doggie wheelchair. But Norman had a lot of dignity and I didn't want to keep him here just for me. I thought about it for days. I prayed about it. I talked to Norman about it. And the answers were all the same. It's time to let him go. His job is done. So on November 22, 2003 a week after the printed book was released and a week before Thanksgiving, I let Norman go over the Rainbow Bridge. I know that he's having fun running and playing again. His spirit is still with me, and I am still grateful to have had him with me the extra 2 years.

Letting him go was the hardest thing I've ever done. I miss him immensely. Not a day goes by, that I don't think about him. But I know it was time, and it was the best thing for him. He was very special and we shared a very strong connection.

It has taken me over two years to put the final updates (about Norman) in this book. Every time I sat down to write it, I would get emotional and then I couldn't get the words out.

Whenever someone mentions the video, it reminds me of how glad I am to have that video of me and Norman. It's priceless. I watch it every so often. It brings back so many memories. It makes me smile, and it makes me cry. I'll never forget my faithful friend.

I am so happy to know that there are other people out there as dedicated to their dogs as I am. Everyone who writes to me, is so in love with their dogs. I think we are a special type of human with a strong connection to our animal friends. They provide us with so much joy and love. The other humans, who don't have this connection, don't know what they're missing.

Please don't let the death of Norman discourage you. Remember he lived nearly 2 years after his initial diagnosis of cirrhosis, even though he was given only a month to live. Plus, I know of other liver dogs who went on to live 3 or more years with liver disease. If anything, please remember Norman as a wise dog who taught us all how to take care of our furry family members. He taught me so much about unconditional love. He is still an inspiration to me. And I hope his life goes on to help thousands of other dogs with liver disease.

With all my hope for your dogs' healing,

Cyndi

Rainbow Bridge

Author Unknown

Just this side of heaven is a place called Rainbow Bridge.

When an animal dies that has been especially close to someone here, that pet goes to Rainbow Bridge.
There are meadows and hills for all of our special friends so they can run and play together.
There is plenty of food, water and sunshine, and our friends are warm and comfortable.

All the animals who had been ill and old are restored to health and vigor; those who were hurt or maimed are made whole and strong again, just as we remember them in our dreams of days and times gone by.
The animals are happy and content, except for one small thing; they each miss someone very special to them, who had to be left behind.

They all run and play together, but the day comes when one suddenly stops and looks into the distance. His bright eyes are intent; His eager body quivers. Suddenly he begins to run from the group, flying over the green grass, his legs carrying him faster and faster.

You have been spotted, and when you and your special friend finally meet, you cling together in joyous reunion, never to be parted again. The happy kisses rain upon your face; your hands again caress the beloved head, and you look once more into the trusting eyes of your pet, so long gone from your life but never absent from your heart.

Then you cross Rainbow Bridge together....

Appendix A: Complete Shopping List

Grocery Store
Protein
Muscle Meat – Whole Chicken or boneless, skinless thighs or breasts, Beef Stew Meat or 85% Lean Ground Turkey or Ground Round

Organ Meat – Chicken Liver, Beef Heart or Beef Liver

Other Protein Options – Tofu, Soy Granules, Fat Free Cottage Cheese, Fat Free Plain Yogurt, Cod Fillet, Free-Range Eggs (no hormones, no drugs)

Complex Carbohydrates (Vegetables)
Fresh Vegetables – Celery, Carrots, Squash, Zucchini

Other Optional Fresh Vegetables - Beets, Kale, Sweet Potatoes, Garlic

Frozen Vegetables – Broccoli Normandy Mixture (Broccoli, Carrots, Cauliflower), Broccoli Cuts, Squash, Baby Peas, Green Beans, Carrots

Canned Vegetables (no-salt) – Artichoke Hearts, Baby Peas, Green Beans, Carrots

Simple Carbohydrates
Pasta, Potatoes, Couscous, Millet or Rice

Spices
Basil Leaves,

Ground Turmeric

Oil
Extra Virgin Olive Oil

Treats and Snacks
Fresh Pineapple Chunks (not canned), Blueberries, Blackberries or Raspberries

Pill-Hiding Food
Prunes, Bananas or Cranberries

Health Food Store
Milk Thistle or Milk Thistle X (150 mg per capsule)

Vitamin E (D-Alpha Tocopherol), 200 IU per softgel capsule

The Missing Link® Dietary Supplement

Other Supplements as directed by your Vet
L-Carnitine (500 mg)

Taurine (500 mg)

Alpha Lipoic Acid (100 mg)

Omega-3 – fish oil/flaxseed oil

Other Remedies that are useful to have around
Homeopathic Remedies - Pulsatilla 6c or 12c (pellets, not liquid)

Bach Flower Remedies – Bach's Rescue Remedy

Specialty Items

Pill Crusher (if giving homeopathic pellets)

Grape seed extract (if giving raw meat)

Veterinarian Items

Digestive Enzymes (Prozymes)

Multi-Vitamin (Canine Plus by Vetri-Science)

Ursodiol (100-150 mg per capsule) prescription

SAM-e (Denosyl) prescription

Appendix B: Healthy Powder

Dr. Pitcairn's Complete Guide to Natural Health for Dogs & Cats gives a recipe for a "Healthy Powder" which contains several important food supplements that should be added to each meal. The Health Powder recipe has been modified for the Sunny's Miracle Diet based on experience and use. Both the original version and the modified version are listed below.

Original Healthy Powder

Amount	Ingredient	Comment
2 cups	Nutritional (torula or brewers) yeast	Rich in B vitamins, iron and other nutrients. (Optional)
1 cup	Lecithin granules	Linoleic acid, choline and inositol, which help your dog emulsify and absorb fats, improving the condition of his coat and digestion.
¼ cup	Kelp powder	Iodine and trace minerals.
¼ cup	Human grade Bonemeal	Enough calcium to balance the high phosphorus levels in yeast and lecithin.
1,000 mg	Vitamin C (ground)	Not required by dogs because they synthesize their own, but personal experiences suggest its value.

Mix all ingredients together in a 1-quart container and refrigerate. Add to each recipe as instructed, usually about 1 tablespoon per meal.

Modified Healthy Powder

Amount	Ingredient	Comment
2 cups	Nutritional (torula or brewers) yeast	Optional
1 cup	Lecithin granules	
None	Kelp powder	Omit kelp to reduce sodium.
½ cup	Human grade Bonemeal	Enough calcium to balance the high phosphorus levels in lecithin.
5,000 mg or 2 tsp	Ester-C (powder)	Ester-C functions as an antioxidant and free radical scavenger, used to repair tissues and protect against cancer, infections, and enhances immunity.

Mix all ingredients together in a 1-quart container and refrigerate.
Add to each recipe as instructed (usually about ¼ tablespoon per meal).

An alternative to this homemade healthy powder is a nutritional supplement for animals with special nutritional needs called The Missing Link®. (see Product Resources)Appendix C: Blank Checklist

	Sunday	Monday	Tuesday	Wednesday	Thursday	Friday	Saturday
Date							
Wake-Up Time							
Medication Time							
Breakfast Time							
Potty Patrol Check							
Medication Time							
Lunch Time							
Ursodiol							
Potty Patrol Check							
Lunch Vitamins							
Medication Time							
Dinner #1 Time							
Potty Patrol Check							
Medication Time							
Dinner #2 Time or Snack							
Potty Patrol Check							
Night Vitamins							
Bedtime Medication Time							
Potty Patrol Check							
Other Notes							

Appendix C: Norman's Case History

PATIENT INFORMATION

Name: Norman
Sex: Male, Neutered
Birthday: 05-05-91
Breed: Cocker Spaniel

Date	Vet	Description of Examination and Treatment	Test Results	Reference Range
1/31/96	RG	Heartgard Green chew 26-50 Program Yellow 21 to 45# (flea)		
5/10/97	RG	**Dental Tarter**		
7/3/98	RG	**Dental Clean & Polish Teeth <50** DHLP/Parvo Annual, Rabies Advantage DOG 2.5ml RED		
10/26/98	RG	**Upset Stomach** Liquipect liquid with Antibiotic Centrene Injection Subcutaneous Fluids		
6/11/99	RG	**Dental Care Recommendation** DHLP/Parvo Annual, Rabies Geriatric Health Profile Rimadyl 75 mg tabs — ½ pill every 12 hours as needed for pain Advantage DOG 2.5ml RED Heartgard Green chew 26-50		
12/28/99	RG	**In Pain** Heartgard Green chew 26-50		
5/30/00		Grooming	**Weight:34.5**	
10/10/00	RG	**Lipoma Left Rib Cage** **Osteoarthritis hip joints** **Patellar Luxation Bilateral** DHLP/Parvo Annual, Rabies X-Ray, Routine Rimadyl Caps 75mg x 60 – ½ tablet 2x/day		
12/09/00 to 12/15/01	RG	Rimadyl Caps 75mg x 60 – ½ tablet 2x/day Heartgard Green 6 Month Supply		

Date	Vet	Description of Examination and Treatment	Test Results	Reference Range
3/30/01		Grooming	Weight:34	
09/21/01	RG	**Gingivitis +++++++** **Sebaceous Adenoma** Tumor Removal DHLP/Parvo Annual, Rabies Torbugesic Inj (for pain) Dental Clean & Polish Teeth <50 **Moderate calculus and tartar build up.** Rinsed mouth with Hexarinse	Weight:28.9 GLU=100.3 **BUN=4.9 (L)** ALT=34 Blood Test **HCT=34.9 (L)** HGB=12.4 MCHC=35.5 WBC=12.6 GRANS=10.0 % GRANS=79% L/M=2.6 %L/M=21% **PLT=165 (L)** Retics=0.6% TP=6.0	76.0—145.0 16.0—36.0 12—130 Ref. Range 37.0—55.0 12.0—18.0 30.0—36.9 6.0—16.9 3.3—12.0 1.1—6.3 175—500 5.70—8.90
		Initial Diagnosis of Liver Disease		
12/15/01	RG	**Listless. Not active. Eating not normal. Polyuric/Polydipsia Left side just behind the ribs a large lump feels like a Lipoma Needle Biop – Just Fat Abdomen feels as if might have some fluid Heart sounds OK Lungs clear** Canine l/d cans STOP taking Rimadyl	Weight: 31.2 Temp: 102.5 General Health Profile **ALB=2.02 (L)** ALKP=103 **ALT=199 (H)** AMYL=1030 **BUN=10.2 (L)** Ca=8.61 CHOL=120.7 **CREA=0.73 (L)** GLU=127.2 PHOS=4.04 TBIL<0.10 TP=5.89 GLOB=3.87	Ref. Range 2.60—3.90 14—111 12—130 500—1500 16.0—36.0 7.80—11.30 110.0—320 0.80—240 76.0—145.0 3.10—7.50 0.00—0.90 5.70—8.90 2.80—5.10
			Blood Test **HCT=36.6 (L)** HGB=12.3 MCHC=33.6 **WBC=17.8 (H)** **GRANS=15.2 (H)** % GRANS=85% L/M=2.6 %L/M=15% PLT=204 Retics=1.3%	Ref. Range 37.0—55.0 12.0—18.0 30.0—36.9 6.0—16.9 3.3—12.0 1.1—6.3 175—500

Date	Vet	Description of Examination and Treatment	Test Results	Reference Range
			<u>Urinalysis</u> Leukocytes=Neg Creatinine=200 Ketone=Neg Blood pH=8.5 Glucose=Neg Bilirubin= + Protein=100 Specific Gravity=1.043 Clear Yellow w/Normal Odor	
12/17/01	RG	Exam & Board Day Only Bile Acid Pre&Post Study	Weight: 31.70 <u>Bile Acids Test</u> **Pre Meal=81.8 (H)** **Post Meal=152.6 (H)**	<u>Normal</u> <13 <25
12/20/01	AV	**Radiographic/Sonographic Findings:** An abdominal ultrasound was performed. The liver was extremely small and difficult to image. The liver was diffusely hypoechoic and coarse in echogenicity. Hepatic mass lesions were not seen. The gall bladder was small. The left medial liver lobe measured approximately 5.8cm dorsoventrally by 2.3cm cranial to caudal. There was a large volume of anechoic fluid present throughout the abdominal cavity. Abnormalities were not seen in the spleen. There was slight decreased coricomedullary differentiation in both the right and left kidneys. Adrenal glands were not visualized. The urinary bladder appeared normal. Gastrointestinal lesions were not identified. Intra-abdominal lymhadenopathy was not seen. There was uniformly relatively hyperechoic mass noted in the cutaneous tissues associated with the left corsal abdomen: this mass was external to the peritoneum. The peritoneum was slightly convex into the abdominal cavity around this mass. This was felt to represent a cutaneous lipoma. **Radiographic/Sonographic Conclusions:** Small diffusely hypoechoic hepatic parenchyma. The possibility of hepatic fibrosis and vaculclar or degenerative hepatopathy should be considered. Moderate volume abdominal effusion. Mild chronic renal changes. **Recommendations:** Symptomatic management for liver failure is suggested. If the patient is non-responsive to medical management or histopathology is desired, an ultrasound guided biopsy could be obtained under heavy sedation/anesthesia. A coagulation profile would be suggested prior to biopsy.		
12/20/01	MH	Phone Consultation **Owner called to say that patient had ultrasound and ultrasonographer found a lot of fluid in the abdomen. Owner was concerned that patient would be in immediate distress because of the large amount of fluid. Told owner that we do not usually drain that fluid unless patient is in immediate distress. Draining fluid decreases blood protein levels.**		
12/22/01	RG	Office Visit, Follow-Up Amoxicillin 250 mg caps 1 tablet 2x/day for 20 days Adequin 0.6 cc 2x/week for 3 weeks, then 0.6 cc 1x/month for arthritis Silymarin 150mg 1 tablet 1x/day to support liver function		

Date	Vet	Description of Examination and Treatment	Test Results	Reference Range
1/05/02	MH	Check-up, follow up blood work **Patient doing much better. Eating l/d well. Abdomen not bloated. Patient on Milk Thistle. Liver enzymes good. Albumin increased.** Continue l/d diet Continue Milk Thistle Start Antioxidants (Vitamin E and selenium) Consider Ursodeoxycolic acid	Weight: 26.80 Temp: 102.00 Blood Test ALKP=79 GGT=4 **ALB=2.43 (L)** ALT=113 (normal)	 Ref. Range 14—111 1—12 2.60—3.90 12—130
1/12/02	RG	Check-up, follow up blood work **Owner complained that Norman is still vomiting, having diarrhea, is still bloated and has a ravenous appetite.** **Norman really seems to be doing well as possible. It seems now the real dx is Cirrhosis of the liver and there is very little else we can really do. A liver transplant only "real" solution.** **Prognosis is poor, only a few weeks to a month.** Increase amount of (l/d) food to 1 ½ can / day Amoxicillin 250 mg caps 1 tablet 2x/day for 20 days Start Ursodiol Tabs 250mg ½ tablet 1x/day for liver disease	Weight: 27 Blood Test ALKP=90 GGT=4 **ALB=2.22 (L)** ALT=91 **BUN=4.4 (L)** **CREAT=0.65 (L)** GLU=108.3 TP=6.17	 Ref. Range 14—111 1—12 2.60—3.90 12—130 16.0—36.0 0.80—2.40 77.0—125.0 5.70—8.90
1/14/02	O	**START DIET – Sunny's Miracle Diet + Ester C, Teeter Creek Liver Tonic STOP Amoxicillin**		
2/11/02	RG	Ursodiol Tabs 250mg ½ tablet 1x/day		

Date	Vet	Description of Examination and Treatment	Test Results	Reference Range
3/9/02	MH	Re-Check Blood Work	Weight: 28	
		Blood work looks good. Recommend Denosyl sd4	Complete Blood ct **WBC=18.0 (H)** RBC=5.8 HGB=12.6 PCV=38 MCV=65 MCH=21.6 MCHC=33	Ref. Range 6.0—16.9 4.8—9.3 12.1—20.3 36—60 58—79 19—28 30—38
			Neutrophils%=71 **Absolute neut=12780 (H)** Lymphocytes%=13 Absolute lymph=2340 Monocytes%=4 Absolute monos=720 Platelet estimate adequate	60—77 2060—10600 12—30 690—4500 3—10 0—840
			Superchem AST=46 ALT=62 T.Bili=0.2 Alk Phos=127 GGT=9 TP=6.3 ALB=2.7 GLOB=3.6 CHOL=122 BUN=18 **CREAT=0.8 (L)** PHOS=3.9 Calcium=10.3 GLU=101 Amylase=741 Lipase=347 Sodium=149 Potassium=4.2 Na/K ratio=35 Chloride=114 **CPK=47 (L)** Triglyceride=69 Osmolality, calculated=310 Magnesium=1.7 Corrected Calcium=11.1	Ref. Range 15—66 12—118 0.1—0.3 5—131 1—12 5.0—7.4 2.7—4.4 1.6—3.6 92—324 6—25 4—27 2.5—6.0 8.9—11.4 70—138 290—1125 77—695 139—154 3.5—5.5 27—38 102—120 59—895 29—291 277—311 1.5—2.5

Date	Vet	Description of Examination and Treatment	Test Results	Reference Range
3/25/02	MH	**Patient vomited all his food last night. Patient was having diarrhea, seems listless and not wanting to eat now.** General Appearance: Quiet Integumentary: Normal Musculoskeletal: Normal Circulatory: No problem noted Respiratory: Normal Digestive: Normal Teeth: WNL Gentourinary: Normal Eyes: WNL Ears: WNL Neurosystems: Good Lymphnodes: Normal Mucous Membranes: Normal Reproductive system: WNL Rule-outs: -- final liver failure -- gastroenteritis IV fluid therapy with B-complex added for the night, if not improved, will do bloodwork. **Patient ate breakfast brought by owner, seemed brighter, will send home.**	Weight: 26 Temp: 101.70	
4/22/02	MH	Ursodiol Tabs 250mg ½ tablet 1x/day		
4/24/02	DF	**Second Opinion** Consultation, exam, and review of history Taurine 500mg 2x/day for liver and cognitive L-Carnitine 500mg 2x/day for liver and cognitive Alpha-Lipoic acid (ala) 100mg 1x/day for cognitive Lower Vitamin E from 400 to 200 IU – d alpha form Double dose of Milk Thistle from 150mg 1x/day to 150mg 2x/day Add Turmeric 1 tsp daily to his food Switch from human vitamin to Canine Plus Multi-Vitamin with antioxidants Switch from human digestive enzymes to Prozyme digestive enzymes		

Date	Vet	Description of Examination and Treatment	Test Results	Reference Range
7/2/02	DF	Patient vomiting and severe diarrhea 1.0 PENICILLIN INJ 1.0 CENTRINE INJ CHEM6 + CBC	General Health Profile ALKP=113 ALT=30 BUN=11.4 CREA=0.70 GGT=1 GLU=106.1 K=4.58 Cl=116.2 Blood Test HCT=46.3 HGB=15.1 MCHC=32.6 **WBC=20.9 (H)** **GRANS=18.7 (H)** % GRANS=89% L/M=2.2 %L/M=11% PLT=287 Retics=0.6%	Ref. Range 23—212 10—100 7.0—27.0 0.50—1.80 0—7 77.0—125.0 3.50—5.80 109—122 Ref. Range 37.0—55.0 12.0—18.0 30.0—36.9 6.0—16.9 3.3—12.0 1.1—6.3 175—500
8/27/02	DF	Comprehensive Exam	Weight: 24.3	
9/10/02	DF	Patient in Pain Re-Check Exam **Torbutrol Tabs 5mg** one every 8 hours for arthritis pain	Weight: 25.5	
9/11/02	DF	Patient crying, acting painful, limping on the back left leg, abdomen is swollen. Temp: 101.6 **Gave 1 torbutrol last pm – caused sedation for several hours then pain seemed to return after meds worn off. Increased anxiety.** Keep for Rads of spine / left leg / pelvis. Rads – Severe proliferation osteoarthritis of both coxofemoral joints. . Luxation (7x?) of right femoral head. Irregular joint surface of femoral intercondylan area (L) – ACL? Severe calcified discs, but do not see evidence of IVD rupture / herniation. Increased gas in stomach / intestinal loops. Returned Torbutrol tabs.		
10/7/02	DF	Re-Check Exam	Weight: 24	

Date	Vet	Description of Examination and Treatment	Test Results	Reference Range
11/11/02	DF	Re-Check Exam	Weight: 25.4	
		Urinalysis and sediment Chemistry (6 panel)	General Health Profile ALKP=78 ALT=30 BUN=14.4 CREA=1.08 GGT=1 GLU=101.0 Na=153.8 K=5.01 Cl=117.8 Urinalysis Urobilinogen=normal Glucose=neg Nitrite=neg Leukocytes=net Ketone=Neg Blood=Neg pH=6 Bilirubin ++ Protein=+/30 Specific Gravity=1.025 Color=Yellow Appearance=Hazy	Ref. Range 23—212 10—100 7.0—27.0 0.50—1.80 0—7 77.0—125.0 144—160 3.50—5.80 109—122
2/11/03	DF	Re-Check Exam	Weight: 24.6	
4/24/03		Grooming	Weight: 24	

Date	Vet	Description of Examination and Treatment	Test Results	Reference Range

5/22/03	DF	Re-Check Exam
		
		CBC + CHEM25
			<u>CBC</u>
			HCT=34.7 (L)
			HGB=12.2
			MCHC=35.2
			WBC=8.4
			GRANS=6.6
			  % GRANS=76%
			  Neut=5.3
			  EOS=1.1
			L/M=2.0
			  %L/M=24%
			PLT=201
			
			<u>CHEM25</u>
			ALK Phosphatease=58
			ALT (SGPT)=59
			AST (SGOT)=36
			CK=82
			GGT=6
			Albumin=2.9
			Total Protein=7.2
			Globulin=4.3
			Total Bilirubin=0.2
			Direct Bilirubin=0.0
			BUN=17
			Creatinine=0.9
			Cholesterol=155
			Glucose=82
			Calcium=10.7
			Phosphorus=3.8
			TCO2 (Bicarbonate)=18
			Chlorine=120 (L)
			Potassium=4.6
			Sodium=152
			A/G ratio=0.7
			B/C ratio=18.9
			Indirect Bilirubin=0.2
			NA/K ratio=33
			Anion Gap=19
			Ammonia=38
				<u>Ref. Range</u>
				37.0—55.0
				12.0—18.0
				30.0—36.9
				6.0—16.9
				3.3—12.0
				
				2.8—10.5
				0.5—1.5
				1.1—6.3
				
				175—500
				
				<u>Ref. Range</u>
				10—150
				5—60
				5—55
				10—200
				0—14
				2.5—3.6
				5.1—7.8
				2.8—4.5
				0.0—0.4
				0.0—0.1
				7—27
				0.4—1.8
				112—328
				60—125
				8.2—12.4
				2.1—6.3
				17—24
				105—115
				4.0—5.6
				141—156
				0.6—1.1
				
				0.0—0.3
				27—40
				12—24
				0—169

"We have many effective and potent drugs available in our armamentarium. As the activity and potency of drugs increased, so has the risk of serious adverse effects. Rational use of drugs includes a consideration for the potential adverse effects, especially serious toxicity, and the ability to recognize adverse effects.

Do not dismiss an unexplained disorder in a patient until a drug-induced cause has been ruled out.

The Greek physician Hippocrates (440 - 375 BC) provided an ethical basis for the practice of therapeutics. He recognized that a physician sometimes does more harm than good.

(This applies to veterinarians as well.)

The advice of Hippocrates, "primum non nocre" (translated: above all, do no harm) reminds us that it is better to administer no therapy at all than to administer therapy that might be harmful."

- Papich, Mark G. DACVCP - (Diplomate, American College of Veterinary Clinical Pharmacology)

Adverse Drug Reactions of Clinical Significance.

The Central Veterinary Conference August 23-26, 2003.

IDEXX VETERINARY SERVICES
Online results at www.vetconnect.com
West Region   800-444-4210
East/Central/Colorado   866-433-9987

512-353-1871   ACCOUNT #: 35261

PATIENT   SNASAL,NORMAN

REQ #: 14008725   LAB #:   D1678904
AGE: 12   SEX: M   COLLECTED: 05/24/2003
SPECIES: CANINE   RECEIVED: 05/24/2003 16:05
BREED: SPAN COCK   REPORTED: 05/26/2003 05:02

DOCTOR: FORSTER

TEST PROCEDURES	RESULTS	REFERENCE RANGE	UNITS
CHEM 25			
ALK. PHOSPHATASE	58	10-150	IU/L
ALT (SGPT)	59	5-60	IU/L
AST (SGOT)	36	5-55	IU/L
CK	82	10-200	IU/L
GGT	6	0-14	IU/L
ALBUMIN	2.9	2.5-3.6	g/dL
TOTAL PROTEIN	7.2	5.1-7.8	g/dL
GLOBULIN	4.3	2.8-4.5	g/dL
TOTAL BILIRUBIN	0.2	0.0-0.4	mg/dL
DIRECT BILIRUBIN	0.0	0.0-0.1	mg/dL
BUN	17	7-27	mg/dL
CREATININE	0.9	0.4-1.8	mg/dL
CHOLESTEROL	155	112-328	mg/dL
GLUCOSE	82	60-125	mg/dL
CALCIUM	10.7	8.2-12.4	mg/dL
PHOSPHORUS	3.8	2.1-6.3	mg/dL
TCO2 (BICARBONATE)	18	17-24	mEq/L
CHLORIDE	120 (H)	105-115	mEq/L
POTASSIUM	4.6	4.0-5.6	mEq/L
SODIUM	152	141-156	mEq/L
A/G RATIO	0.7	0.6-1.1	
B/C RATIO	18.9		
INDIRECT BILIRUBIN	0.2	0-0.3	mg/dL
NA/K RATIO	33	27-40	
ANION GAP	19	12-24	mEq/L
AMMONIA	38	0-169	ug/dL

SNASAL,NORMAN   *** FINAL REPORT ***   PAGE 1 OF 1

Tickle-Blagg Animal Hospital
1100 Highway 80
San Marcos, TX 78666
512-353-1871

Species : Ger Canine >8yr
Patient : Norman
Client : Cyndi Smasal

Ver: 6.9
Date : 22-May -2003 02:18PM

Test	Results	Reference Range	Indicator
			LOW NORMAL HIGH
HCT	= 34.7 %	37.0 - 55.0	
HGB	= 12.2 g/dl	12.0 - 18.0	
MCHC	= 35.2 g/dl	30.0 - 36.9	
WBC	= 8.4 x10⁹/L	6.0 - 16.9	
GRANS	= 6.4 x10⁹/L	3.3 - 12.0	
%GRANS	= 76 %		
NEUT	~ 5.3 x10⁹/L	2.8 - 10.5	
EOS	~ 1.1 x10⁹/L	0.5 - 1.5	
L/M	= 2.0 x10⁹/L	1.1 - 6.3	
%L/M	= 24 %		
PLT	= 201 x10⁹/L	175 - 500	

Buffy Coat Profile

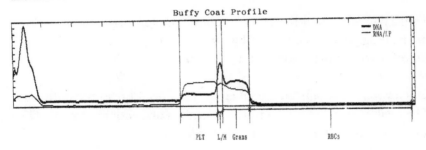

PLT   L/M Grans   RBCs

95

Appendix D: Quick-Start Guide

This Quick Start Guide has been written to help your dog get on the road to healing. I'm sure you're worried about your dog. You're looking for some quick answers. You don't know if this will really work. You don't know where to start.

I'm about to hand you the abbreviated version of the alternative treatment I used to heal my dog Norman. This newly designed Quick Start Guide has been written to guide you through the initial crisis when your dog is first diagnosed – letting you get started today!

These pages contain the exact information you need right now to get the healing process started. I'll walk you through the critical first steps. I'll refer you to page numbers in the book for further information.

Once you're through the initial crisis, you should read the entire book. The healing process for liver disease is not a one shot treatment. There's a lot more to it than what's in this guide.

So get ready: I'm going to go through this information quickly, step-by-step, to give you the specific actions you'll need to get through this critical stage of liver disease.

Step 1 – Gather Data

1) What symptoms are present?

Vomiting
Diarrhea
Eating unusual things
Frequent urination or accidents
Drinks a lot of water
Depression or lethargy
Stopped eating
Very hungry
Orange urine
Pale gray stools or orange/yellow stools
Jaundice – the whites of the eyes, skin and gums turn yellow.
Lost weight
Gained weight
Swollen belly filled with fluid
Behavioral changes: seizures, aimless pacing or circling, head pressing, acting needy
Unexplained bleeding or prolonged bleeding
Bad breath
Strong "dog" odor or bad smell

2) What are the test results? (How bad and how far along?)

- Blood Test Results for liver disease, end stage liver failure, cirrhosis
    High Liver enzymes (ALT , AST, GGT)
    Bile Acids
    Bilirubin
    Low Cholesterol
    Low Potassium

- Ultrasound
    Small Liver
    Enlarged Liver
    Mass in Liver
    Shunts on Liver
    Scar Tissue
    Percentage of Liver affected: _____
    Cancer
    Abscesses
    Abnormal Blood Supply
    Gall Bladder
    Bile System

- Biopsy
    Condition of Liver Cells
    Apparent Cause

3) What is the prognosis?

Less than a week
One to two weeks
Less than a month
Three to six months
Over six months

4) What is the diagnosis?

None
Liver Disease
Cirrhosis
Hepatitis
Other: _____

5) What is the history?

Vaccinations
Blood Tests
Medications
Heart Worm control medications
Flea & Tick control medications
Steroid treatments
Pain treatments
Seizure treatments
Surgery
Infections
Dental Problems
Dental Cleaning
Digestive Problems
Arthritis
Arthritis treatments
Genetic ailments
Other

6) What is the treatment?

None
Medications
    Antibiotics for infections
    Anti-Inflammatory - Steroids
    Liver Support - SAM-e
    Bile System - Ursodiol (form of bile)
    Water Retention – Lasix
    Digestive Aid - Pepcid
    Others
Stop taking harmful medications
Diet
    Same
    Prescription Diet
    Natural or healthy homemade diet

Supplements
    None
    Liver (Hepato) Support (Milk Thistle and others)
    Antioxidants – like Vitamin E
    Others
Treat Symptoms
Treat the Whole System

Step 2 – Where to Start

If your dog has blood test results with high liver enzymes:

…Start by giving your dog Milk Thistle and Vitamin E in the following dosages:
- Milk Thistle - 100mg per 25lb, 2 times a day
- Vitamin E – 200 IU per day

Then read Chapter 1 and Chapter 2 to understand liver disease and this alternative treatment.

If your dog has four or more of these symptoms, and high liver enzymes:

Common Symptoms:
- Vomiting with or without blood.
- Diarrhea with or without blood.
- Eating unusual things.
- Frequent urination and increased water intake.
- Depression or lethargy – doesn't want to play anymore, lays in a spot away from you and family.
- Loss of appetite or ravenous appetite.
- Orange urine.
- Pale gray stools or orange/yellow stools.
- Jaundice – the whites of the eyes, skin and gums turn yellow.
- Chronic weight loss or wasting.
- Ascites - swollen belly filled with fluid.
- Severe neurological signs - behavioral changes, seizures, aimless pacing or circling, head pressing. (May be associated with mealtime.)
- Unexplained bleeding or prolonged bleeding (e.g. after nail trimming or drawing blood).

…In addition to Milk Thistle and Vitamin E, give your dog:

- Vitamin B complex – 50mg 2 times a day
- Canine Plus Multi-Vitamin with Antioxidants (or 1/2 of human Multi-Vitamin per day)
- Distilled water instead of tap water for the first 4 weeks, then use spring water

Then read Chapter 3 and Chapter 4 to learn how to develop a healthy diet for treating liver disease.

If your dog is taking Antibiotics, Steroids or any other Anti-inflammatory medications:

…Stop or quickly taper off these harmful medications. In addition to Milk Thistle and Vitamin E, add Omega-3 Fatty Acids to provide Antioxidants, Anti-Inflammatory support, and help liver, joint, and brain functions.

Of course, check with your Vet about the right dosage for your dog and ask about starting additional supplements listed in Chapter 5.

Again, make sure you read Chapter 3 and Chapter 4 to give your dog the food that heals the liver.

If your dog is taking Heart Worm or Flea control medications:

…Stop giving your dog these medications and do NOT give your dog any Vaccinations. Then review the list of other items to avoid found at the end of Chapter 5, and make necessary changes.

Again, make sure you give your dog Milk Thistle and Vitamin E to remove harmful toxins and improve liver function. As well as read Chapter 3 and Chapter 4 to give your dog a healthy diet.

If your dog is NOT eating:

...Start by reading Chapter 3 to get ideas on what type of food is good for your dog, then proceed to Chapter 4 for recipes to start with. Try to find anything in these chapters that your dog will eat.

Once you've found the type of food your dog will eat, you'll be ready to begin creating your own recipes. Review Chapter 1: "Norman's Next Crisis..." and "Trial and Error..." sections. These sections will help you learn how to identify food items to avoid.

Then read Chapter 7: "Gastritis or Stomach Problems" to better understand common stomach problems. Look for clues to identify the underlying cause and appropriate treatment. A digestive aid like Pepcid might be needed to treat the upset stomach before your dog will begin to eat again. Add digestive enzymes to each meal to aid digestion. Add slightly cooked potatoes or yams to each meal to remove toxins from the bowels.

In addition to Milk Thistle and Vitamin E, give your dog Vitamin B complex to stimulate the appetite. If your dog is taking Antibiotics or SAM-e these may cause nausea and lack of appetite. Stop giving your dog these medications to see if they are causing the appetite problem.

However, if you still can't get your dog to eat over the next 2-3 days, you should see your Vet to determine why and avoid dehydration.

If your dog is Hungry all the time:

...Start by reading Chapter 3 to get ideas on what type of food is good for your dog, then proceed to Chapter 4 for recipes to start with. Make sure you are feeding your dog enough food in multiple small meals. If you are only feeding your dog two or three times a day, add another small meal either at night before bed or in the middle of the day.

Then evaluate the amount of protein you are putting in each meal. Slowly add more protein to each meal. Of course, be sure you are giving your dog top quality sources of protein like: soy, fat free cottage cheese, fat free yogurt or top grade boiled meat.

Again, make sure to give your dog Milk Thistle and Vitamin E to improve liver function.

If your dog is vomiting (at night or in the morning before eating):

...Start by reading Chapter 3 to get ideas on what type of food is good for your dog, then proceed to Chapter 4 for recipes to start with. Find a recipe that your dog will eat.

Once you've found or created your own recipe. Review Chapter 1: "Norman's Next Crisis..." and "Trial and Error..." sections. These sections will help you learn how to identify problem foods.

Then read Chapter 7: "Gastritis or Stomach Problems" to better understand common stomach problems. Look for clues to identify the underlying cause and appropriate treatment. A digestive aid like Pepcid might be needed to treat the upset stomach. Add digestive enzymes to each meal to aid digestion.

Ask your Vet about your dog's Bile System and if additional bile is needed to help with digestion. Your Vet will need to give you Ursodiol (or other form of bile) or a prescription to get it from a pharmacy.

Step 3 – Care for Your Sick Dog

While your dog is in crisis, your love and attention are some of the most important factors in your dog's recovery. Here are the critical areas that need your attention.

1) Good Veterinary Care

Now is the time to discuss alternative treatments, diet and supplements with your Vet. During the course of treating liver disease, you will be seeing your Vet on a regular basis. Make sure you will get the type of treatment you need and the answers to your questions.

2) Watching symptoms and looking out for signs of getting worse

At this critical stage of liver disease things can change for the better or for the worse. Watch your dog like a hawk. Review Chapter 6 "Communication from Your Dog" to learn what to look out for. Take notes and track your dog's progress.

3) Potty Patrol

Your dog's stool is a major indicator of health and a diagnostic tool. Get in the habit of watching your dog potty. Notice the amount, color, consistency, odor (if unusual) and frequency of your dog's stool. Review Chapter 6 "Potty Patrol" and "What diarrhea tells you about your dog" to learn more about what each of the above indicators tell you about your dog's recovery.

4) Signs of Progressing Liver Disease

If the original symptoms do not go away, and the following symptoms appear, the liver is not responding or there could be other problems.

- Depression or lethargy
- Swollen Belly (Ascites)

- Jaundice (yellow eyes, gums, and skin)
- Chronic Weight Loss

Review Chapter 6 "Signs of Progressing Liver Disease" to learn more about each symptom. Then go back and read the rest of Chapter 6 to learn more about caring for your sick dog.

Of course, check with your Vet if any of these symptoms appear.

5) Take care of yourself

Your dog's health is affected by your emotions and mental state. So it is very important that you tend to your own mental and physical health.

- Stay positive and eliminate as much stress as you can from your life.
- Be as relaxed, confident and as calm as possible.
- When you are upset, avoid interacting with your dog.
- Take breaks and rest when you need it to gain a fresh perspective.

Review Chapter 6 "Emotional Health" to learn more about how your emotions affect your dog. Then go back and read the rest of Chapter 6 to learn more about caring for your sick dog.

Step 4 – Check Results

The purpose of taking notes, tracking progress and checking blood levels is to increase the chance of a full recovery. Symptoms and blood levels will tell you whether the treatment is making things better or worse. Frequent blood tests give you feedback to make adjustments right away if the treatment is not working. It also gives you comfort and encouragement when things are getting better.

- Your Vet will run weekly or monthly blood tests to track progress
- Your note of symptoms and stool indicators will tell you when to get further treatment from your Vet
- Your regular examination will monitor your dog's overall health and track progress
- Your note of behaviors, diet and appetite will help you identify food problems

Read Chapter 6 "How to Give Your Dog a Quick Check-up" to learn about other health indicators.

Of course, this step is on-going. In the beginning you will check results more frequently. But later, as the treatment progresses and the crisis ends, you will perform these check-ups less frequently.

Important Note: Do not use this guide as a substitute for reading the book or treatment by a veterinarian. Rather, use this information to get through the initial crisis in conjunction with veterinary care. Once you are past this crisis, go back and read the entire book. This is only a summary of the alternative treatment.

Conclusion

Inspiration to put together this Quick Start Guide came from previous *Hope For Healing* book owners. While I continue to hear positive reports about alternative treatment and information that I share in my book, I know that many of you sometimes feel overwhelmed and don't know where to start. It's feedback from people like you that's compelled me too put together this Quick Start Guide.

I want to be absolutely certain that you have all the information and resources you need to care for the dog that you love....including the benefit of my personal guidance in the form of this Action Plan.

I pray that you have as much success as I have. I encourage you to ask your Veterinarian questions and do your own research. Don't give up without trying. And, take good care of yourself and your dog. You'll feel better knowing you did everything you could to care for, save or prolong you dog's life.

Resources and References

Products

1) Canine Plus by Vetri-Science Multi-Vitamin is only available from a Veterinarian. If your Vet does not carry Canine Plus try one of these: http://www.catvitamins.com/consumers.html

2) Liver Tonic by Teeter Creek Herbs, http://www.teetercreekherbs.com/formulas/lvrtone.html

3) Sojourner Farms Dog Food Mix, http://www.food4pets.com/sojofood/sojdogfood.htm

4) Halo Spot's Stew For Dogs, http://www.petfooddirect.com/store/product1.asp?pf_id=20212501KT1

5) Hydrolyzed Lactalbumin Protein (whey protein), http://www.wellvet.com/lactalbumins.html

6) The Missing Link® by Designing Health, http://www.designinghealth.com/products/canine_products_main.html

Bibliography

1) Messonnier, S., Natural Health Bible for Dogs & Cats, Prima Publishing, 2001

2) Pitcairn, R., Pitcairn S., Dr. Pitcairn's Complete Guide To Natural Health for Dogs & Cats, Rodale, 1995

3) Schultze, K., Natural Nutrition for Dogs and Cats, Hay House, 1998

4) Yarnall, C., Natural Dog Care: A Complete Guide to Holistic Health Care for Dogs, Journey Editions, 1998

5) Griffin, J., Carlson, L., Dog Owner's Home Veterinary Handbook 3rd Edition, Howell Book House, 2000

6) Yeager, S., The Doctors Book of Food Remedies, Rodale, 1998

7) Balch, P., Balch, J., Prescription for Nutritional Healing 3rd Edition Avery, 2000

Other Sources

1) Aleithia Artemis, Author and Animal Behavior Specialist and long-time studier of health-related influences. http://www.topnotchtraining.net. 713-PAW-PETS. Email: TNT@TopNotchTraining.net.

Articles used as References

1) Dr. Fleming, "Liver Disease: Signs, Symptoms, and Diagnosis," http://www.geocities.com/Heartland/Plains/1151/LiverDisease.html

2) Dr. Michael T. Murray, "Nature's Liver Remedy: Milk Thistle Extract," Ask the Doctor

3) Decker Weiss: NMD, AACVPR, "Liver Health – Milk Thistle," Ask the Doctor

4) Chocolate Chip Creations, "Pets Need Wholesome Food Also – A Hassle Free Guide to Wholesome Natural Pet Food," http://www.pet-grub.com

5) The Senior Dogs Project, "A Review of Signs of a Potentially Life-threatening Reaction to Rimadyl," http://www.srdogs.com/Pages/rimadyl.ade.steps.html

6) Kennalea B. Pratt, "Sunny's Miracle Diet," http://www.minschnauzer.com/diet/sunny.html

7) W. Jean Dodds, DVM, "Dr Dodd's Liver Cleansing Diet," http://www.canine-epilepsy-guardian-angels.com/liver_diet.htm

8) Janet Tobiassen Crosby, DVM, "How is a Bile test performed, and what does it mean?" http://vetmedicine.about.com/od/diseasesandconditions/f/FAQ_bileacidtst.htm

Canine Liver Disease Resources

1) Yahoo Group - Canineliver-d, dedicated to the support of owners of dogs with liver disease. This list is for owners of dogs who currently have or have had dogs with some type of liver disease. This can range from infectious hepatitis survivors to Porto systemic shunts to chronic active hepatitis. This list is mainly for support of the owners not for providing the type of medical advice a Vet can provide. Each case is individual and the treatment for liver conditions is complex so what is true for one may not be true for another dog. To join send email to: canineliver-d-subscribe@yahoogroups.com o

2) Nation Wide Laboratories – Test Interpretation General Notes. A technical guide to blood test results. http://www.nwlabs.co.uk/testinterpindx.html

3) Long Beach Animal Hospital – website dedication to Liver Disease. Includes easy to read explanations and helpful picture illustrations. http://www.lbah.com/liver.htm

4) Information from Dr Michael Richards on Liver Disease in Dogs. http://www.vetinfo4dogs.com/dliver.html

5) An overview of Liver Disease - http://www.vetevents.com/news/articles/46.html

6) Liver Disease Signs, Symptoms, and Diagnosis - http://www.canine-epilepsy.com/liverdisease.htm

More Resources

1) Search for a Holistic Veterinarian in your area at the AHVMA (American Holistic Veterinary Medical Association) - http://www.ahvma.org/referral/

2) Q&A about Liver Disease in Dogs http://www.vetinfo4dogs.com/dliver.html

3) Understanding Your Pet's Blood Work http://www.cah.com/library/labtests.html

About Norman

05/05/91 – 11/22/03

Norman was not my whole life,
but he made my life whole.

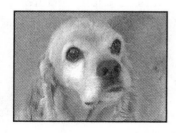

John "Norman" City-Slicker Smasal an AKC registered Cocker Spaniel born May 5th, 1991. He weighted around 24 pounds, had big brown eyes, and silver buff hair. He loved to sing, especially "Happy Birthday". His favorite pastimes were playing with his buddy, taking naps, eating treats, chasing Calvin the cat, and going for car rides to San Antonio to visit Cyndi's parents and their 3 dogs (Amber, Jarrett, and Avery). He graduated with honors from Rob Carey Training School with his Basic Training degree.

You can see him on video with Cyndi when they lived at their home in Wimberley, Texas.

http://www.hopeforhealing.com/NormanVideoMed.wmv

About the Author

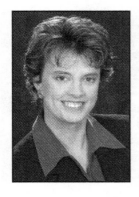 **Cyndi Smasal** successfully cared for her "liver dog" Norman for two years after his initial diagnosis. She is an Internet Marketing Mentor/ Coach who shows other entrepreneurs how to start a business online. Cyndi has a Bachelor of Science degree in Computer Science from the University of Texas at San Antonio. Before becoming a professional marketing coach, Cyndi worked in the high-tech computer start-up world, where she spent 15-years in the Software Quality Assurance field. Now, she's a trained professional coach from the Coach Training Institute, and a Certified Guerrilla Marketing Coach. She lives in Austin Texas.

Cyndi Smasal

http://www.cyndismasal.com

CPSIA information can be obtained
at www.ICGtesting.com
Printed in the USA
LVHW091037170521
687618LV00021B/172

9 781434 319166